Mouths of Babes

MOMOSA
PUBLISHING

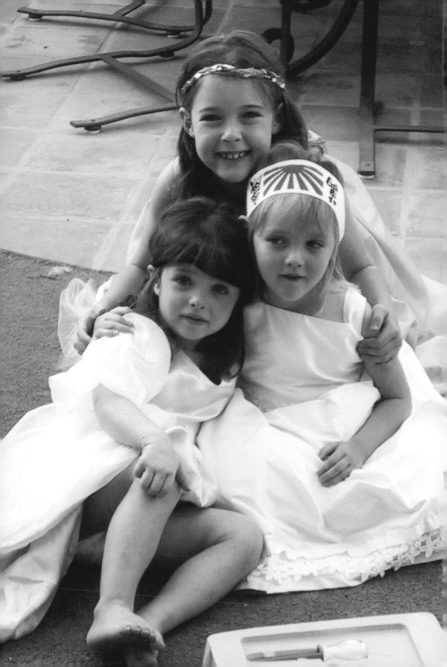

Mouths of Babes

Everything I Learned in Medicine, I Learned from My Kids

Susan S. Wilder, MD

Printed in the United States of America

Cover and interior design by Joanna Williams

Library of Congress Control Number 2017909909

ISBN 978-0-9986531-8-1

2 4 6 8 10 9 7 5 3 1 paperback

Visit our parent company at MomosaPublishing.com

To all the moms, dads, and doctors
who never feel enough—love is always enough.

Introduction

●●

Practicing medicine and parenting have much in common. Both are "practices," perpetual works in progress where perfection and balance are illusory. They are both as much arts as they are sciences. Parenting and doctoring are both humbling, awe-inspiring, exhausting, and profoundly rewarding. Both provide moments of sheer panic and instances of supreme exuberance, tears and laughter, frustration and exhilaration. Both require similar tools: resilience, extreme diligence, perpetual patience, humility, and an incontrovertible sense of humor. Years of sleep deprivation and grueling self-sacrifice are part and parcel of both.

They say the military is the "toughest job you'll ever love." I have experienced that arena, too, but the military does not hold a candle to medicine or parenting.

I often observe that my children arrived on this Earth to keep me humble. As a physician with a typically atrocious work schedule, I was never that mom who met them at the school bus with freshly baked cookies, nor was I often the one who tucked them in at night. However, because I was blessed with a supportive husband and an excellent nanny, my "Mommy time" was pure, unadulterated quality. Because my time with my kids was so priceless, I treasured every second. Although I was remiss at video- and photo-documenting my children's lives—though we have about a thousand pictures of our first daughter's first week of life—I did keep a book of "-isms," capturing the adorable comments, witticisms, and fractured aphorisms of my girls' early childhoods. I often quote these endearing quips because they contain precious pearls of wisdom that apply to everyday life. A friend of mine coined them "witty wild Wilder women words of wisdom!"

I have also found my girls' witticisms to be astonishingly relevant to the practice of medicine. That's what inspired this book. I hope that aspiring doctors, physicians and other healthcare providers find these words, filtered through my experience, helpful as we evolve as healers and as parents.

I hope you enjoy these bits of wit and find a dose of comfort, appreciation, humor, or insight within.

Acknowledgments

I am eternally grateful to my parents for their unconditional love, for their "Greatest Generation" wisdom borne of overcoming hardship, and for the gift of an incomparable education that I enjoy paying forward every day. My parents also gave me a huge family full of love, support, and occasionally a necessary dose of humility.

To all of the patients in my career who honored me with their most important asset—their health, I am profoundly grateful. You challenged, supported, questioned, comforted, and taught me every day to be a wiser physician and a better human being.

My appreciation is boundless for my husband, Bob, my self-appointed "accommodator," whose support gives my dreams wings, nurturing and making them even grander than I ever imagined. We are proof positive that opposites do attract. The pure synergy of our complementary skills and natures makes everything we do together exponentially better.

And, last but not least, to the three amazing women we are blessed to call daughters, your dazzling spirits never cease to amaze and inspire me. Your staunch independence, which honestly was often challenging to parent, assures me that you will forge your own paths without constraint. Your empathy, sense of fairness, and perpetual kindness make me believe our world is safe in your capable hands. Your sarcasm and humor assure me you will always enjoy the gift of laughter—the best medicine. Of all the titles and accolades bestowed upon me over my career, the title of "Mom" will always be my most cherished.

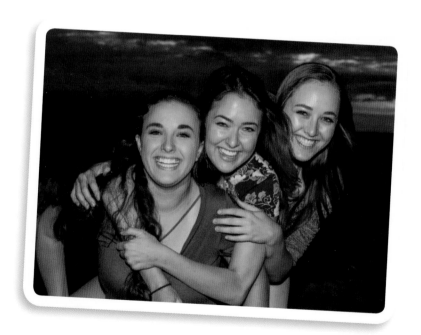

> ## Once at first you don't **exceed**, try, try again.

This adorably fractured aphorism so perfectly illumi-
nates American culture. We excel at over-indulgence.
The majority of our chronic disease, disability, and prema-
ture death are caused by excess—over-eating, over-imbib-
ing, over-working, over-stressing, over-medicating, and
over-dosing on "busy-ness" and electronics to the detri-
ment of sleep, true social connections, and exercise. We are
even "over-doctored!" While our diseases of excess keep me
in business, an emphasis on resuscitating endangered
concepts of *moderation* and *discipline* deserves our utmost
attention.

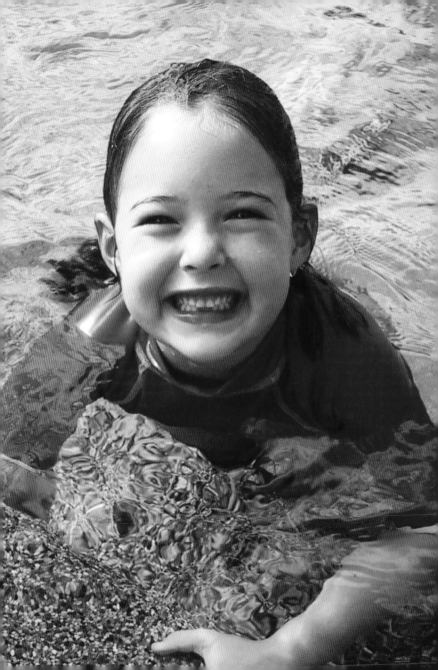

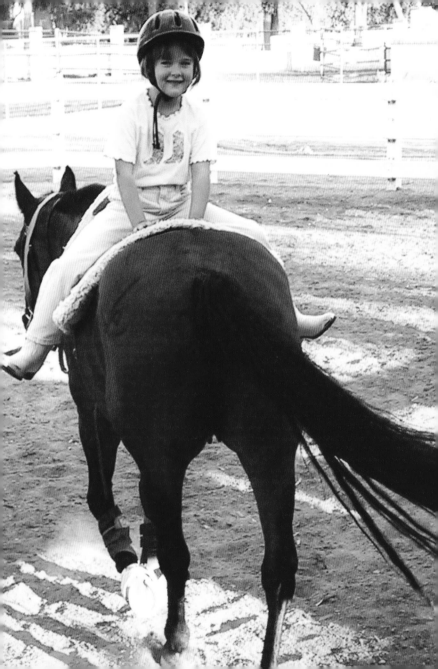

Sometimes people just do crazy things!

Over more than a quarter century as a family physician, I have learned that human beings are neither rational nor logical. We are predominantly emotional. This truism allows me to better understand the roots of the irrational, unhealthy choices all people, myself included, make every day. In my decades as a medical educator, I often observed physicians in training get frustrated with "noncompliant patients" and often give up on them. However, as motivational speaker and author Tony Robbins once noted, "You cannot influence someone while judging them." Physicians would do well to understand that changing people's behavior is not our job. We must endeavor to inspire, empower, and shine a light of reality, guiding patients (or our children) toward making better choices, head over heart, more often. From this lesson came the mission of Lifescape Premier: "Inspire Health," because we cannot create health.

I'm not whining;
I'm suggesting!

My children are brilliant negotiators, as are many of my patients. My parents' generation, who traversed the Great Depression and World War II, rarely complained but rather just pulled their own bootstraps and solved problems. Whining was an unaffordable luxury. Complaining rarely gets us anywhere, yet it is a pernicious reality of our entitled culture. As a parent, business owner, and physician, I try to deflect complaints and instead seek ideas for solutions. Patients mired in "victim mode," who complain incessantly about their circumstances, are beyond help. Guiding people to get out of their own way, past limiting beliefs that shackle them to perpetually failed outcomes, is the most challenging and gratifying work we do.

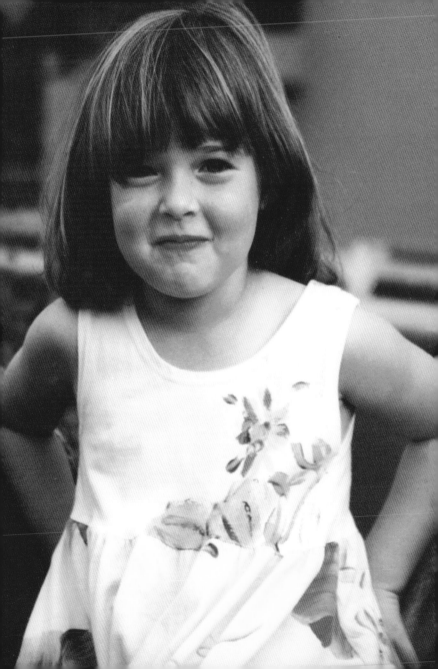

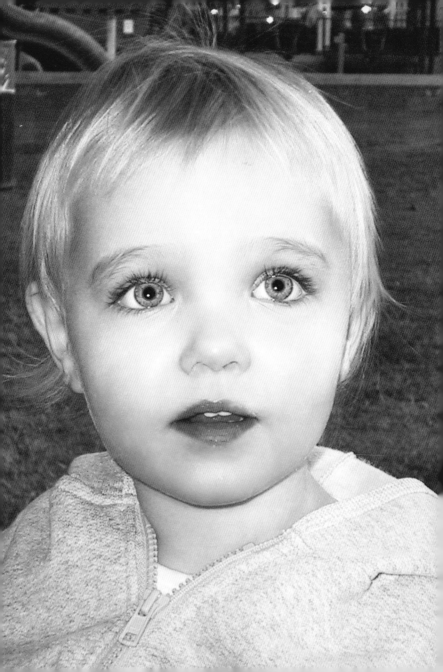

I don't want to know about sad things.

Nobody wants to face the sad things in life—like death. However, it is an absolute certainty that each of us will. My friends thought I was crazy taking my kids to visit dying patients in hospice. I taught my children that dying is a natural part of life and dying people deserve comfort and companionship. In all honesty, my adorable little munchkins were far more therapeutic than I would ever be! We earn resilience by facing hardship. Protecting our kids or our patients from hardship robs them of those critical lessons and the resilience that grows from having endured and overcome. As physicians, one of our most important tasks is to help patients face sad things, plan for scary eventualities, and voice their own wishes. Facing our mortality inspires us to treasure the incredible miracle of human life.

> ## I a little scary (in the dark). My eyes are broken, and I can't see myself!

We all have fears; some of us to the point of extreme phobia. Most of those fears are just our minds running amok in a negative direction. I like the phrase "seeing in the dark" as a metaphor for facing the demons of irrational thoughts and learning to challenge and handle them. Here's an example: A visit with a hypnotherapist convinced a patient to "decide" that his horrific nerve pain, which failed to respond to every conventional therapy, was just an annoyance and not really painful. Another patient dropped her high cholesterol 100 points by working with a therapist to "release worry." Opening our minds and our hearts to see differently can yield surprising results in transforming health. Though as someone once said, "It's okay to have an open mind, as long as it's not so open that your brains fall out." The more I know, the more I realize how little I know. The art part is learning to heal while negotiating the dark unknown. No wonder they call medicine a "practice."

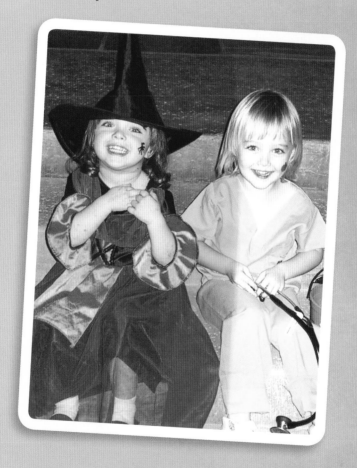

Mouths of Babes

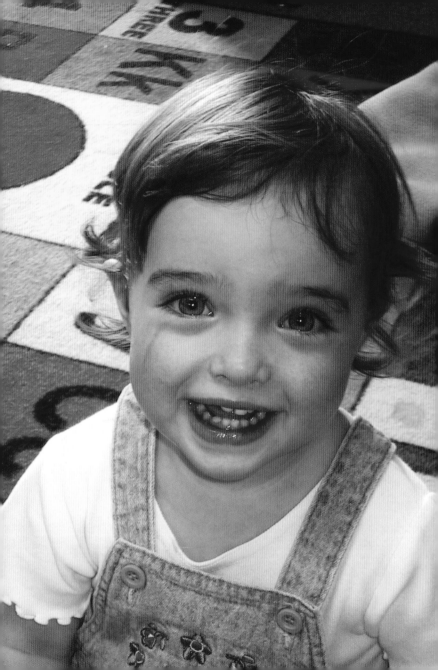

It's okay; sometimes mommies make mistakes, too.

I grew up believing I had to be perfect. However, my children and my work as a physician rapidly taught me that perfection is not achievable and in *no* way desirable. The cost of perfection is evident in the extreme breadth of human suffering we face—depression, anxiety, insomnia, eating disorders, chronic fatigue, drug and alcohol abuse, and even overdose and suicide. The price of perfection is exorbitant, and physicians suffer these issues at much higher levels than the general population. I am convinced that the only thing worse than being a perfectionist is having one as a parent, teacher, or doctor! Allowing ourselves to be vulnerable, admit our failures, and embrace our imperfections are wonderful gifts to give to ourselves, our children, and our patients.

Why should I cover my mouth when I cough? What if I don't want to keep it?

When my daughter uttered this witticism, I had no comeback! Her logical argument made perfect sense, but it reminded me that we do not live in a vacuum. For example, when parents choose not to vaccinate their children, I explain the role of vaccines is to protect ourselves, but also to protect the most vulnerable in our community. I could not live with myself if I didn't vaccinate my child, and then my children's pregnant teacher, their newborn cousin, an aunt undergoing chemo, or an asthmatic friend died. It will be a very sad day if we adopt a completely selfish mindset of "it's only about me" rather than "all for one and one for all." Divided, we fall.

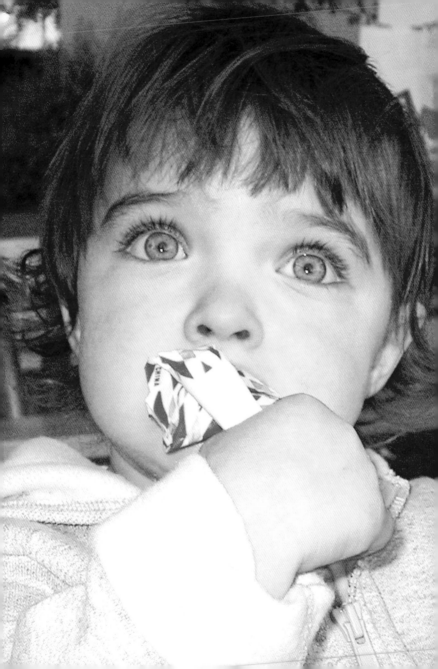

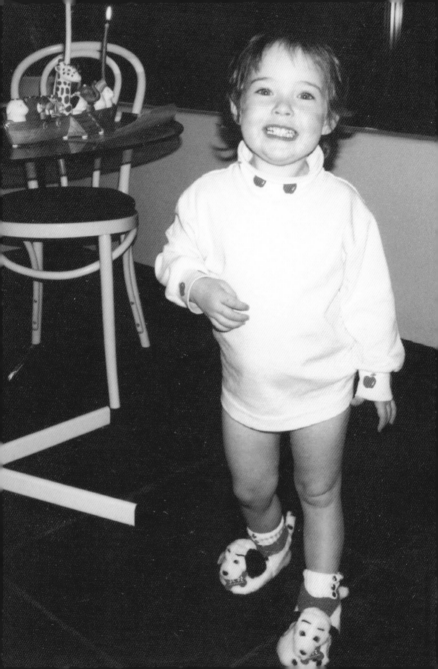

> I don't feel so bad
> being Jewish anymore
> 'cause there's a kid in
> my class who has
> diabetes!

Perception is powerful. Insecure bullies target people who are different from themselves—whether the difference is skin color, clothing, religion, hair, body type, socioeconomic status, or mental or physical health conditions. A parent once publicly shunned my daughter with eczema because she feared her child would "catch that *awful ugly* rash!" One of my dear elderly patients was bullied in the dining room of her luxury residence when other diners claimed to be "disgusted by her tremor," which caused her to spill food on occasion. I pray for the day when we all appreciate and tolerate the differences in each other and learn to treat each other with kindness and compassion. There but for the grace of God…

They look sad;
we should smile them!

Just paying attention and tuning in to the feelings of others is intensely powerful medicine. Even when there is nothing more to do clinically, we always have the capacity to comfort. Empathy, however, can be a blessing and a curse. Sympathizing with the struggles of others is always healthy, but truly feeling and taking on the discomfort of another is fraught with danger. Maintaining healthy clinical boundaries depends on tamping down the desire to fix and please everyone. However, doing our best to bring a smile to others, particularly those who are struggling, harnesses the very best of humanity. Our most challenging patients (and children) are often the ones who need our unconditional love the most.

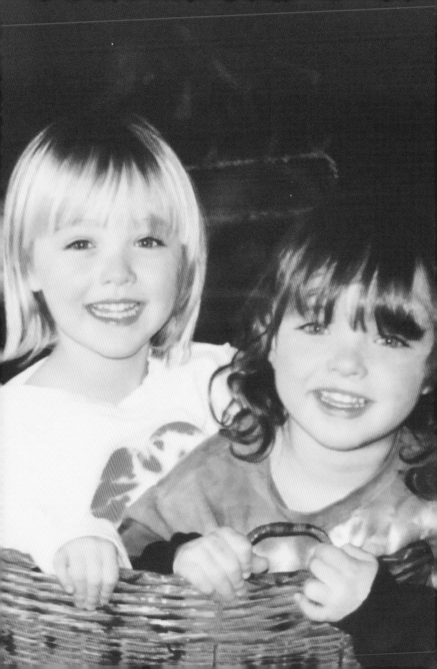

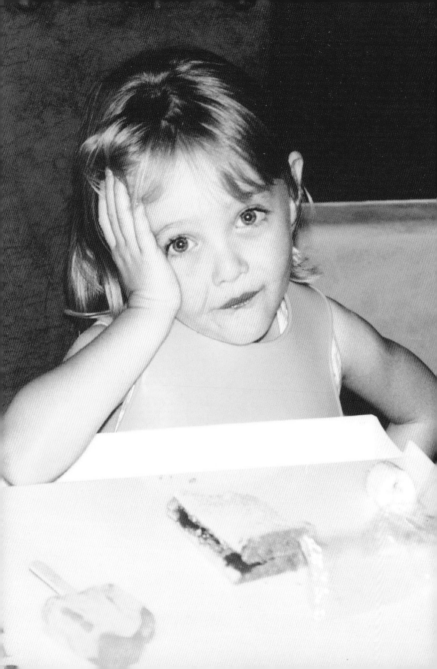

> # I'm especially good at procrastination, but I haven't gotten around to it yet.

Patients often delay their annual physicals or lab testing, noting, "I haven't been good," to which I reply, "I'd rather see truth than fiction!" How often do we procrastinate about our health? "I'll start that diet after the party," or "I'll begin exercising—again—on New Year's." One of my patients even lamented, "If I had someone cook all of my meals and make me exercise, I'd be fine." What happened to discipline? Too often, health hits the priority list only after we lose it. Our healthcare system excels at rescue, while prevention receives less than 3 percent of the healthcare dollar. Our most critical task is convincing patients to focus proactively, and not procrastinate, on their health. As one put it, "Without health, there is no life, liberty, and pursuit of happiness."

I'm not talking back; I'm barguing!

Our patients, like our kids, do not always fully buy into our recommendations. Patient care must be a collaboration. As I often taught medical students: Our jobs are to guide, inspire, and empower patients to make healthier decisions for themselves, not to *change* behavior. One of my favorite "barguing" situations was with a patient whose alcohol intake was verging on risky, with worrisome health consequences. When abstinence was rejected as an option, I suggested limiting intake to less than five ounces per night, to which she gleefully countered with, "Of tequila?!?" Oh yes, "barguing" is a wonderful facet of human nature.

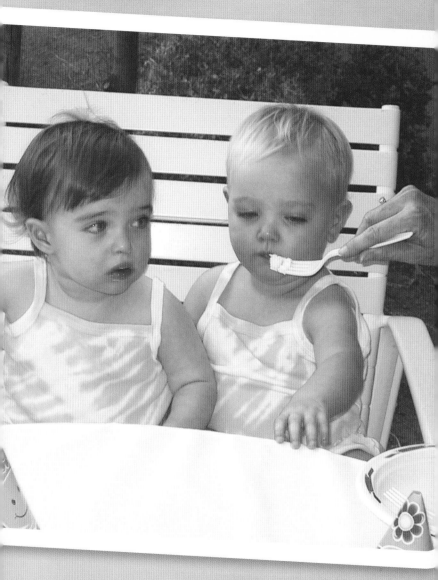

Mouths of Babes

> Sticks and stones may break your bones, but words hurt more than anything.

Words have tremendous power. In medicine as in life, we often wield them carelessly. My husband taught our kids, "Words are like hands. They can build, create, and comfort, or they can injure, harm, and destroy." I spend countless hours deprogramming patients encumbered with persistent negative thoughts, such as, "I have *severe* attention deficit, so I'll never be successful," or "My spine is a *train wreck*." Well-intentioned medical providers often carelessly plant negative comments, sentencing patients to negative mindsets and negative outcomes. You get what you focus on. So if our intent is to inspire healing, then we need to use positively focused words such as, "You have incredible resilience, and I am certain you can work with physical therapy to overcome your injury," or "Here are the positive attributes of attention challenges and a list of highly successful people who have harnessed them to their advantage." How much suffering could we avert simply by using more care in our language, in our families, healthcare, education, business, and politics? As the beautiful aphorism attributed to Buddhism teaches, "Let your words pass through three gates: Is it true? Is it kind? Is it necessary?" And I would add, "Is it constructive?"

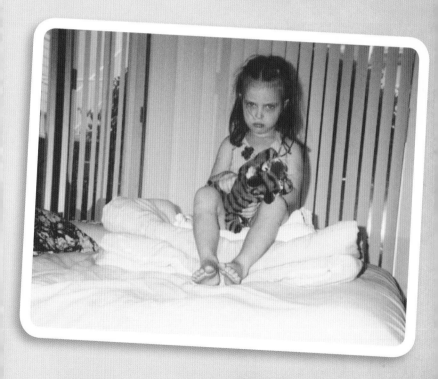

Mouths of Babes

> # "We made breffast all by ourselves . . . we eat the marshmallows all gone!"

Unhealthy food options abound, and instant gratification is compelling, no matter our age or stage. The amount of chocolate I consumed while penning this simple tome is astounding, and I rationalized every bite! Sugar can be addictive, causing a brain rush not unlike that of cocaine. The vast majority of children, my own included, consume more than twice the recommended amount of added sugars every day—bad Mommy! I've seen well-meaning moms bring giant cupcakes, packed with a week's worth of saturated fats and sugars, for "snack" for young kids! When my daughter expressed this witticism, it was a reminder for me to break the addiction cycle and get addictive sugar-laden foods out of the house. If it's in the house, it's in the mouth.

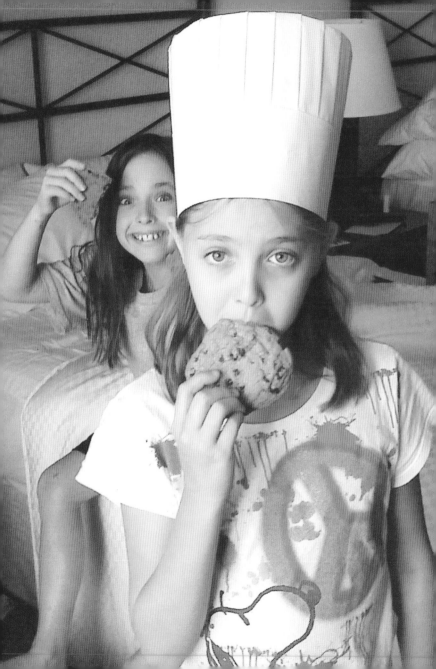

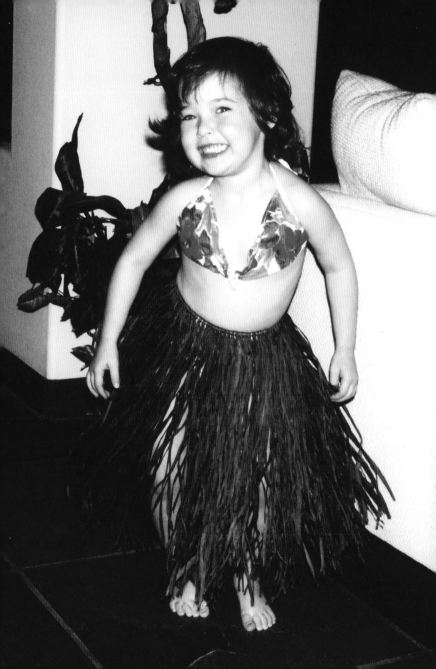

"Mom, your boobs are out of air!"

My response, "That's why they call it *a bust*, honey." We raised our kids in Scottsdale, Arizona, which I lovingly dubbed "the *silicone* valley" because enhancements are so prevalent, it is unusual to see a natural set. No wonder my child thought I was the anomaly! Media portrayals, particularly of women, fuel body-shaming, and they also promote a plethora of unhealthy medical consequences—from anorexia and bulimia to suicide. Kids as young as five experience shame and sometimes bullying about their appearance. Teens are getting plastic surgery at record rates. I never allowed women's magazines—or anything that made me feel inferior—into my home, but the Internet unavoidably inundates us with unhealthy perceptions. Are our kids hearing us talk about dieting, cellulite, or those love handles we hate? Are we encouraging patients to focus on fitness or fatness? Learning to love ourselves unconditionally, including our imperfections, and modeling the same for our patients—and also for our kids—is a gift that pays tremendous rewards.

Mommy, why you put that 'messed up' on your face?

Good question! I often get preachy about eating organic, buying wild-caught seafood and grass-fed beef, and avoiding toxic chemicals in the home. However, like most women, I probably apply more than 100 unproven and potentially toxic chemicals to my body and face before I get out of the bathroom every morning! Research links endocrine disruptive chemicals to some of the most significant scourges we face, including autism, attention deficit disorder, obesity, diabetes, Parkinson's, and Alzheimer's disease. Health is a work in progress for all of us. From the mouths of babes, this statement made me thoughtfully reevaluate the habits I was practicing and modeling for my children. Do as I say, *and* as I do!

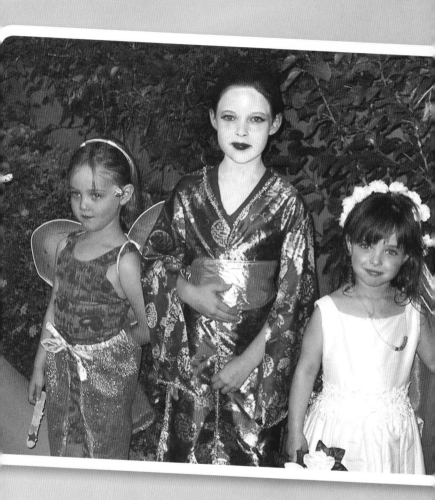

Mouths of Babes

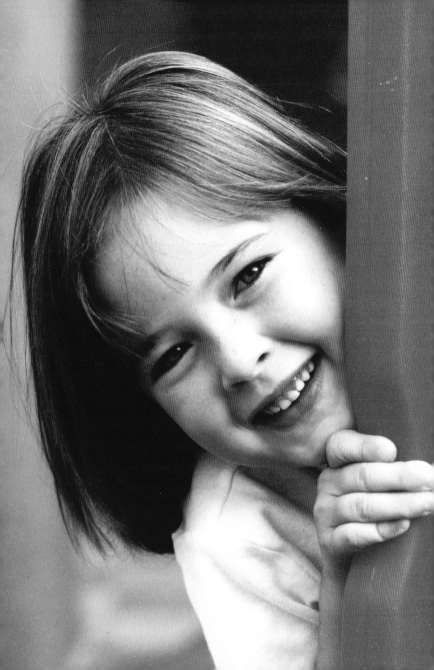

Stop obstrupting me!

We all have basic human needs to be heard and understood. Yet the distractions of our overscheduled lives impede real listening. The incessant pressure to see more patients in less time while fielding exponentially more complex issues and options is a prescription for disaster. Studies reveal that physicians interrupt patients within 23 seconds of sharing their stories. Imagine how frustrating that must be for patients! The time pressures of hit-and-run insurance-centered medicine are a lose/lose scenario both for the patient and for the provider.

We also "obstrupt" by throwing prescriptions at symptoms, the expedient solution, rather than getting to the root causes of patients' issues. We enable patients' disabilities by pretending our drugs are appropriate shortcuts around the lifestyle choices that would really transform their health. For me, shifting to a direct medical practice, working directly for patients, eliminating the insurance middleman, ended our "obstrupting" and opened the door to patient-centered, proactive, comprehensive medicine.

"I understand; I just don't understand."

How often do we admit our ignorance? How often am I really sure my patients, or my kids, understand what I am asking or expecting of them? I find medical students often go through a hazing process in training, and they are often bullied into hiding their ignorance. A physician who is afraid to admit, "I don't know," is extraordinarily dangerous. In medicine, as in life, the more I learn, the more I realize how little I know. I often caution my students, "If you ever think you know it all, you better get out of this business." It is equally important for parents to model vulnerability, imperfection, and the ability to admit our own limitations by looking things up, getting more training, or asking for help.

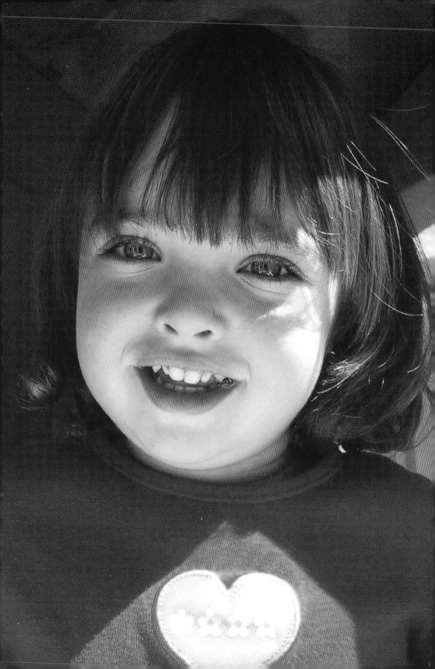

> # I'm a little bit bad and about the middle of good.

This truism perfectly describes every one of us! Helping patients make small steps toward health, without being derailed by "being bad," is critical in healthcare. Taking an all-or-nothing approach is doomed to fail. Shooting for the achievable goal of "a little more good and a little less bad" is a strategy that's much more likely to be successful, especially if we vigorously celebrate the wins.

Every medical intervention we offer is honestly "a little bit bad and about the middle of good" as well. We tend to oversell the medications we prescribe. But, in reality, many medicines work just marginally better than placebo—the power that an intervention can heal purely by virtue of the belief in its healing ability. Truthfully, every intervention we offer has the *potential* to heal, to suppress a symptom, to harm, or to do absolutely nothing—but drain the patient's wallet!

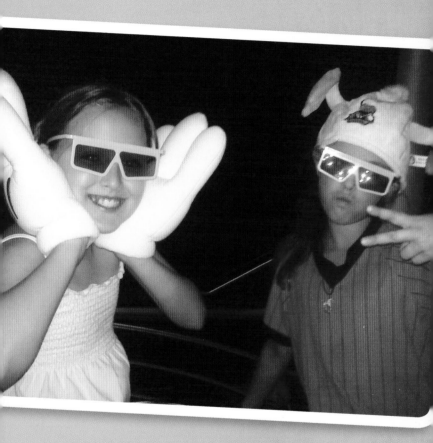

Mouths of Babes

About the Author

Family physician Susan Wilder, MD, co-founded two revolutionary practices dedicated to proactive health transformation. She began her career in the U.S. Air Force where she deftly juggled breast pumps and chemical warfare gear. She served 14 years in academic medicine, including directing the Family Medicine Residency at Mayo Clinic Arizona. Dubbed a "medical maverick" for her frank, insightful, thought-provoking views on healthcare, she is a prized healthcare consultant, national speaker, and media guest. She served as a consultant to DreamWorks Television on the medical reality show "Miracle Workers."

Concierge Medicine Today lists Dr. Wilder among the "Top Doctors in Concierge Medicine" nationally while the Consumers Research Council and Best Doctors lists her among the nation's top Family Physicians. She is a multiple recipient of Phoenix Magazine's "Top Doc," 101 North Magazine's "People's Choice," Arizona Foothills Magazine's "Best of our Valley," and Ranking Arizona's "Best Family Doctors" awards. Dr. Wilder received Arizona Business Magazine's "Health Care Leadership Award," Phoenix

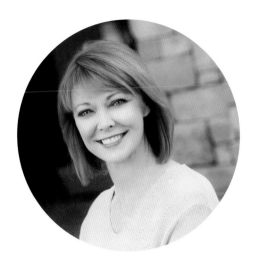

Business Journal's "Outstanding Women in Business," and Greater Phoenix Chamber of Commerce ATHENA finalist. She even earned a tiara as eWomenNetwork's "Mom Entrepreneur of the Year."

She studied meditation with Deepak Chopra, brain health with Dr. Daniel Amen, human motivation with Tony Robbins, and Functional Medicine with Dr. Mark Hyman. Dr. Wilder grew up in Honolulu, Hawaii, the sixth of seven siblings. She attended Punahou school with a young Barak Obama, does a lovely hula, surfs poorly, and was a triathlete until blindsided by a wayward golden retriever. Dr. Wilder met her husband on her first day of college. With 3 kids and a business to run, their parenting philosophy blended benign neglect and whatever works. Dr. Wilder finds respite in inspirational books and quotes. When not working (never), Dr. Wilder enjoys hiking, yoga, healthy cooking, and singing to the car radio. She is passionate about inspiring health.

A portion of the proceeds donated to charities involved in children's wellness including:

Healthy LifeStars – inspiring kids for life to be active, eat right, and know they can do it! **www.healthylifestars.org**

ChildHelp USA - prevention and treatment of child abuse. **www.childhelp.org**

Gabriel's Angels – pet therapy for abused kids. **www.gabrielsangels.org**

Boys and Girls Clubs – empowers young people to reach their full potential. **www.bgca.org**

Mothers Awareness of School Age Kids – engage, educate, empower. **www. maskmatters.org**

Digital Citizen Academy – prevention & education for students & educators. **www. digitalcitizenacademy.org**

Touch & Go

Touch & Go

SAM Mc AUGHTRY

THE
BLACKSTAFF
PRESS

BELFAST

● A BLACKSTAFF PAPERBACK ORIGINAL ●

Blackstaff Paperback Originals present new writing, previously unpublished in Britain and Ireland, at an affordable price.

ACKNOWLEDGEMENT

'The Words Are In My Heart' was composed by Harry Warren and Al Dubin and published by B. Feldman and Company Limited; 'That Lovely Weekend' was composed by Moira and Ted Heath and published by Chappell International Music Publishers.

First published in 1993 by
The Blackstaff Press Limited
3 Galway Park, Dundonald, Belfast BT16 0AN, Northern Ireland
with the assistance of
The Arts Council of Northern Ireland

© Sam McAughtry, 1993
All rights reserved

Typeset by Textflow Services Limited

Printed by The Guernsey Press Company Limited

A catalogue record for this book is available
from the British Library

ISBN 0-85640-503-5

AUTHOR'S ACKNOWLEDGEMENT

I would like to acknowledge with gratitude the financial help of the Arts Council of Northern Ireland.

I am grateful also to Robert Bell of the Linen Hall Library, and to various friends in the legal profession for research and advice concerning the legal aspects of this work.

My gratitude goes, too, to my good friend Terry Rogers, of Dublin, prince among turf accountants and world poker authority, who gave me bed space, work space, eating space, and the solitude needed to crack this novel.

ONE

DOWN IN THE CENTRE of Belfast, only twenty minutes'
walk away, the Court of Criminal Appeal was
hearing my case. For some reason nobody had told me that
I wasn't going to be there. For the next two days the
courtroom would be full of men with wigs and gowns and
nothing in their heads but disputation. They would play
the legalistic game, read from law reports, spectacles on
the ends of their noses, determining whether this strand of
evidence should be accepted or that one rejected. It didn't
seem right that they should do this without my being there,
to see and to be seen. It might help to remind them of
just what it was they were about.

Two and a half days and then I would know. Months ago, through all the preliminary appearances and through the trial itself, I had made for myself artificial horizons beyond which I had taught myself not to look, one for each of the early court hearings, one for the trial, one for the appeal, one for the decision of the Minister of Home Affairs as to whether or not he saw any reason to interfere with the due course of the law, and then, of course, only one horizon would be left.

At the end of my trial I had taken the sentence well. The papers had all said so. 'With composure', that's how they'd put it. But when, in two and a half days, they would come to tell me the outcome of the appeal, when I came to the limits of that horizon, there wouldn't be any reporters to tell how I'd take it. I could react in any bloody bastarding way I felt like reacting. It wouldn't matter to anybody except myself.

I should have paid more attention when the lawyers were setting out to me the grounds of my appeal. If I had, I'd have been better able to mark the long hours. As it was, all that I could do was listen to one screw of the deathwatch saying the Serenity Prayer, the boozers' doxology: 'God grant me the serenity to accept the things I cannot change, the courage to change the things that I can, and the wisdom to know the difference.'

It was all right for him – he was going home when his four hours were up, he could look for serenity and courage and wisdom and feel the wife's leg at the same time. But over in England, in a pub called Help The Poor Struggler, Albert Pierrepoint, the public executioner, would be reading about me. I knew all about him. In another world, at another time, Dicky Walters had told me, and Dicky had studied Pierrepoint the way Newton had studied gravity.

2

The hangman was a wee man, liked to sing Irish songs and do conjuring tricks in the bar. If – when – the Court of Criminal Appeal rejected my submission, it would give me three clear Sundays and then I would take a walk. The day before the execution, Pierrepoint would arrive at Crumlin Road jail with his bag. In the bag would be the straps, the rope, the shackle, and the white cap.

When the time came for the wee cunt to slip the white cap over my head, my eyes would have looked on the last horizon.

T W·O

HE BOAT TRAIN FROM Larne slowed just by Jennymount
Mill. Mother had worked there as a weaver before
she'd married Dad. She'd always been proud of it. Weaving
was clean work, not like spinning or doffing; weavers
didn't stand in water with their skirts hoisted up to the
houghs.

My poor, lovely mother was the reason I was here.
Twenty-four hours earlier I'd been in Bari, Italy.

'I say, Reilly, may I?' The C of E padre was a nightly
piss merchant. Life was funny: he could preach Christianity
with a hangover and a clear conscience, while I, an atheist,
felt as guilty as sin about my boozing.

4

I nodded him into the office. When my flying was over they'd made me a staff officer at Air HQ Bari, helping the Eyeties re-form their Regia Aeronautica.

The padre shimmered in, like Jeeves. 'I'm afraid it's not good news, Paddy.'

I was in no condition to hear bad news. It's something I've said to some brass hat last night, I thought. Christ, maybe I've insulted the air vice-marshal. As usual, my sweat seemed to stink like sewer seepage.

'It's your mother, and I'm sorry to say she's seriously ill.' He squeezed my arm. Padres are great touchers. 'Deeply sorry.'

To be truthful, all I'd felt at first was relief. Drink blackouts begot daymares. Only a couple of weeks earlier, on Christmas morning, I'd woken up to learn that the previous evening I'd bopped a fellow officer. He'd disputed my version of 'The First Noël'.

'She didn't say anything in her letters' was all I could say.

'Well, mothers don't, bless them.'

At least with an excuse like this nobody could blame me for beering it up. But they didn't give me time to do it at Bari. When a staff officer was posted away the air vice-marshal liked to have a word, but in my case there was no invitation. It was Johnny Watson, the camp commandant, who said goodbye: 'Mind yourself, Hugh. I'm sorry about your mother.'

Mind yourself.

I'd got used now to my real friends telling me to mind myself. Johnny Watson was fair-haired, blue-eyed, a public schoolboy pilot, going for the law when he was demobbed. We were close, having been squadron buddies. Afterwards Johnny had saved my bacon a good few times on the HQ campus after piss-up balls-ups.

He smiled and shook my hand. 'Just bloody take it easy, you old bugger. You made it through the war – don't cock it up in civvy street.'

He'd got me priority all the way to London. I was on a Communications Flight Anson to Pomigliano in two hours, and fixed up in a Dakota to Blackbush after another two. A day in London, strangely sober, sipping half-glasses of beer like an Englishman, walking into Cox and King's Bank to draw the first pounds sterling I'd seen for three years. The soft-eyed woman in the bank smiled at me. 'I do all the air force officers' accounts beginning with R and S. I know all my officers. So glad that you got through all right.'

The train, groaning and squealing, drew into York Street station. I grabbed my cases, swung down on to the platform, and walked quickly towards the barrier, one of a crowd of returning soldiers, sailors, airmen and merchant seamen, with their suitcases and their kitbags, their wary eyes, and their thoughts. Relatives, friends, sweethearts, waited on the other side of the barrier. Women were crying, being lifted, swung around, feet off the ground; fathers, brothers, shaking hands.

I saw our Bill, in his dungarees. He put out a hand, but when I came up to him I laid my cases on the ground, put my arms around him, and it was touch and fucking go for crying.

He was seventeen, with a face more innocent than mine ever was. He took a case, we went out of the station, past the taxis with the gasbags on their roofs, on to York Street. I pointed Bill towards the Edinburgh Castle on the other side of the road. Halfway there we were halted by a convoy of heavy carts coming up from the deep-sea docks nearby, the huge draught horses striking sparks from the granite square setts.

The road cleared and we crossed to the bar. Inside, in the just-opened smell of disinfectant, Brasso and whiskey, I ordered a short for myself and a mineral for Bill. We sat down beside a soldier in web equipment. I smiled and looked Bill over. His hair wasn't as dark as mine, more of a brown than a black. His eyes were blue and wide and innocent; mine were brown, after Mother's side. He reached up to about the bottom of my ear. When I'd joined up six years earlier, he'd only been four hands higher than a po.

I thought of all the things I'd done that he hadn't. When he was twenty-five he wouldn't be needing the whiskey, for one thing. But it was gorgeous to be home. Bill was looking at me as if I was Gregory Peck. He took a sip of sarsaparilla. 'Flight lieutenant pilot,' he said. 'Tommy Boyd's brother's only a sergeant cook.'

'Up Tommy Boyd, then, with a wire brush.' I sank the whiskey, pretended to punch him on the button, and rose to go.

Walking up Duncairn Gardens, I looked around at the city I'd left behind three years earlier, in January 1943. The blitzed ground between houses was overgrown with weeds and wild grass, and moss had softened the tops of the broken walls. Civilians walked past with their heads down, the women in headscarves and tight-pulled winter coats, the men in grey or brown raincoats and duncher caps. They walked like a people who had lost a war.

'How's Mother?'

Bill didn't hesitate. 'She's very serious.'

It was the first time I'd really thought about her since I'd heard the word from the padre. She was often out of sorts, but seriously ill was a bit much.

Right through the war, she'd written to John and me once

a week. If there were other letters, Mother's was opened last. I loved her, but there was never anything very interesting in a letter from a mother, except maybe the catalogue of casualties among the guys who'd grown up with me. When her weekly letter had stopped about eight weeks earlier I'd hardly noticed.

On the other hand, I had written to her and to Bill just about every other day since February 1940, when I'd enlisted. Mother used to tell me in her letters how much she and Bill looked forward to them. 'If your daddy was here he would be so proud of you, a pilot. I keep all your letters,' she'd say.

Writing letters was a compulsion with me. I had kept up contacts with other aircrew mates, as well. The educated ones never knew that by their letters they were educating me, sparking up my writing, lending to it the shine that Mother had liked so much.

'John's home, too,' Bill said.

Lovely. Bloody lovely.

'He has no good word for you, Hugh. Never had, and he hasn't changed.'

'That doesn't surprise me.'

We turned the corner of the street, and the two old Nesbitt dames were at the door. I'd forgotten about them, the Nesbitts, small and lonely, living their lives at the front door, one on a stool, the other leaning, arms folded, against the doorpost. Maudie, the elder sister, pointed as we appeared, and she and Agnes made squeaky noises of surprise and welcome. I took Agnes's hand and made to do the same with Maudie, but she held me at arm's length and peered up at me. 'You went away a boy, Hughie, but you've come back a man that's seen too much,' she said.

Bill had knocked the door and Maudie was kissing me when it opened. It was John.

'Huh. The Brylcreem boy's home.'

With one glance he took an inventory, from top to toe. I could have done with a haircut; my tunic was wrinkled, the buttons tarnished. I needed a shave; my shoes were muddy and neglected. He gave another snort: 'The Household Cavalry!' He turned away. No handshake, nothing. I followed him up the narrow hall, with its creaking, sagging floor. The joists and doorframe had never been the same since the 1941 air raids. In the tiny kitchen I felt oversized and awkward. Dropping my case beside the other one just inside the parlour, I hung my greatcoat over the banister. Before I had time to do anything else John called me: 'You'd better come up.' He was halfway up the stairs, looking down impatiently. I fell in behind him. He was in army undress, khaki shirt, trousers, and white canvas braces. Barrack-square creases angled through his broad backside; his boots had a high, bullshit shine.

Aunt Nellie, Mother's sister, was waiting outside the back bedroom. She kissed me, held me close, then she let me go and backed towards the front bedroom, out of the way.

John spoke round the door of Mother's room: 'Hugh's home, Mother. He's here.' His voice was soft. With a jerk of the head I was invited to go in.

A low-watt bulb shone weakly through an orange-tinted shade; yellow morning light filtered through an off-white paper blind, three-quarters drawn. The room was set for a dying. It was full of the scary-sweet bedpan smell of the deathbed.

The double bed filled most of the room. I walked around the end of it on the lino, past the tiny hearth, marking the places where Dad used to land his burning Woodbine butts.

Mother, in a pink flannel nightdress and a woollen bed jacket, lay against high-heaped pillows. Her hair was soft, pinned back loosely. I dropped to my knees beside her. She was so weak that she couldn't turn her head towards me, only her eyes moved, and I bent over her, to make it easier.

Her eyes were so sunken that the lids seemed to rest above them, out of contact. The skin was clapped tight to her skull. What had once been wrinkles were now lines drawn on parchment.

I kissed her brow. It felt hot and dry. Her hands rested on the turned-down sheet and I took one in mine. She no longer had a bosom.

Aunt Nellie had come into the bedroom. She stood, with John, at the door. She was Mother's younger sister and she looked as Mother had looked the day I'd left to go overseas – strong black hair, going grey, rolled-up sleeves, energy and bounce in every line of her. 'There now, Betty,' she said, 'that's Hugh home, too. They're home to see you, your two lovely boys. And Hugh's an officer and all.'

The lips fell back from the putty face; I had to bend to hear Mother's voice. 'Aye.' It was a whisper, fighting to get out of a sigh.

'Hello, Mother.' I felt the stick fingers move in my hand. They searched along my own fingers, then came the voice again.

'Your ring?'

'It's downstairs. I was washing myself and left it on the mantelpiece.' As I spoke I looked up. Bill had joined the others, but it was to John that my eyes went. His contempt was clear, for the lie about the ring.

10

I stood up. The bedclothes had fallen away from her and I took the edge of the sheet to draw them up, but John's voice stopped me: 'Watch it, for heaven's sake, she's in agony, can you not see that?'

I straightened, kissed her again, and followed John and Bill. Again I had the cloddish, clumsy feeling as I went back downstairs. I had forgotten how small the house was. The feel of it hadn't come back to me yet.

Down in the kitchen I undid my tunic, hung it in the hall. Aunt Nellie handed me tea in one of the best china cups: Mother's wedding present. The cup rattled and shook so much in my hand that some of the tea spilled into the saucer. I set them on the carpet and lit a cigarette. John and Bill and Aunt Nellie were watching.

It was the woman who showed understanding, as I felt the sweat break. 'You must feel strange, back home again, after three years.'

I nodded, tried lifting the saucer again and made it. As I drained the tea I could feel John's eyes going over me.

'What kind of job were you doing at Air HQ?' Bill asked. He was ready to commit the details to memory for transmission at Canning Street corner that night.

'I was helping the Eyetie air force to re-form,' I told him.

'Bunch of bloody ice-cream sellers,' John growled. 'They were about as much good in the field as a troop of the Girl Guides.'

'Actually, their pilots weren't that bad,' I said. 'It took a lot of nerve to fly some of the out-of-date kites that they had. Our fellows were knocking their SM 79s out of the sky with no bother, and their fighter pilots in the Machi 202s were no joke. They got a good few of ours.'

'All the same, it's great, you being an officer and all,' Aunt

Nellie was smiling shyly. 'It should help you to get a good job when you come out of the air force.'

'I'll tell you one thing,' Bill said, enjoying John's chagrin, 'you'll not be going back to working in Short's.'

I had been a paint-sprayer in the aircraft factory, but when war came I walked out. I just smiled at Bill and looked around the kitchen, at the china cabinet that was new, the scrubbed, bare table and the worn sofa that had been there for as long as I could remember, at the stool that Dad had made, and the four worn and scarred chairs around the table. The lino and rug were new.

Just when she'd begun to clear the house of the war's shabbiness and lift her heart with some new items, Mother was going to die.

'What does the doctor say?' I asked Aunt Nellie, knowing the answer already.

She shook her head as she spoke. 'There's no betterment for your mother, Hugh ... ' She dropped her head and wrung her hands. ' ... No betterment at all.'

I went into the parlour to unpack. There was a brand-new suite of furniture in the room, some sort of fawn tweedy material; scatter cushions lay on the two chairs and the sofa, with larger cushions. A dark carpet had been laid, and over it a light fawn long-haired rug. Beside the door was another new china cabinet. In this, and in the one in the kitchen, were Mother's most loved possessions, two china sets, an EPNS tray, trinkets and souvenirs of bygone trips with the Mothers' Union, the swimming medals Dad had won as a young man, some cheap glasses, a decanter that had never seen wine or spirits, framed photographs of my grandparents, on both sides. There was a new bookcase, empty of books, beside the cabinet. On the mantelpiece two wooden elephants stood sentry, beside each was a brass candlestick, and in the centre was a clock with Westminster chimes.

The parlour was looking nice.

It was a rotten time for her to die. She was only fifty-nine.

THREE

————

D AD HAD DIED IN thirty-eight, earning John promotion
to head of the house. If the game had been straight,
John ought really to have been the officer now, and I the
sergeant. His army blouse, pressed immaculately, was hanging in the hall. His ribbons included the European Theatre
Star, with the tiny oak leaf of a Mention in Dispatches. John
had had a hard enough war in the Ulster Rifles. And he was
still the same, it didn't seem to have taken a pick out of him,
compared to me. But sure that was the way of things in the
air force I'd just left behind. With the shooting over, all the
other fliers I knew seemed to have settled down no bother.
While me? I was still waiting for the other shoe to drop.

I took out the presents: a delicately worked jade brooch from Tunis for Mother, a Spitfire model for Bill, made over many weeks from a piece of copper piping by one of our mess servants in North Africa, an Eyetie POW. There was nothing for John and nothing would be expected. There'd been no direct contact between us for six years. I'd tried writing to him a couple of times through the war but he'd never answered.

There was no trinket or keepsake for Aunt Nellie either, but that would be easily fixed. I brought the presents into the kitchen, set the brooch in a place of honour in the china cabinet, handed the Spitfire to Bill and putting my arm around Aunt Nellie, I led her out to the yard. Closing the door behind us, I took her hand and folded her fingers over two ten pound notes. She tried to give it back, but she had five kids. She kissed me, and then a peep at the amount of money made her hug me, her cheeks rosy with pleasure. Shortly after, she went out.

In the kitchen John was sitting the wrong way round on a chair. 'Hey, Brylcreem, tell me this: what does an orange fabric strip on the ground mean?'

I looked at him blankly.

He repeated it. 'A strip of cloth, long, coloured orange, laid out on the ground. What does it mean?'

Bill's eyes were begging me to give the right reply.

'I don't know what you're talking about,' I told him.

John turned in triumph to Bill: 'What did I tell you?' Then to me: 'It's what we used to spread out to stop you stupid bastards from bombing us.'

I was sitting on the sofa, less than a foot from him. 'Look,' I said, holding myself back from jabbing a finger into his chest, 'I flew a bomber. I flew it at night. At eighteen thousand feet. Over Italy, and Yugoslavia, and Romania, and Austria. That's what I did in the war. The whole of southern Europe could have been one long orange strip and it wouldn't have mattered a monkey's fuck to me.'

Bill's eyes were shining. A round of wild applause looked to be a near thing.

John, on his feet, swung the chair out of the way. 'Who the hell do you think you're talking to?' He was white, and tight-lipped.

I stood up, turned away from him to stop the trembling, looked into the mirror, and began to unbutton my shirt. I rubbed my chin, went into the parlour and came back with my shaving kit.

'You watch it, boy,' John said, his voice rough with anger.

I went past him into the scullery, propped my mirror against the window, and gave myself a cold water shave. My head felt as big as a melon, and my face and lips had that numb and rubbery feeling that comes from travelling through the night. After shaving, I filled the basin with cold water, went outside, bent over the grating, and emptied it over my head.

Back in the kitchen, finishing towelling myself, John said: 'By the way, boy, where is your ring? That was a right load of balls you told my mother.'

She'd given us identical gold rings when we'd enlisted. Mine lasted until mid-1944; I'd missed it from my finger only half an hour after leaving the bed of a cabaret dancer in Naples. I was in an army truck on my way back to Foggia by then. I could never have found my way back to the house in a million years.

'It came off my finger when I was swimming at Rabat,' I told him. 'It was always too big.'

'Like your head.'

I was happy to let it be.

Aunt Nellie came back and went straight upstairs. I got down to polishing my shoes and shining the belt and buttons of my tunic. I had just signalled Bill to go out with me when Aunt Nellie called from the bottom stair. John and I followed her up.

Mother was lying up on the pillows with her eyes half closed. Her breathing was so shallow that it hardly moved the bedclothes. I couldn't watch; I turned and went downstairs.

Her face was nothing like my mother's. The lips were pale and narrow, and above the upper one was a faint moustache; her skin was the skin of an old woman. The woman in the bed looked like an ailing eighty-year-old who had never been bonny and buxom and bouncy.

Kiss, kiss: she was always kissing us. 'Kiss, kiss,' she used to say when we were setting off to school. The least excuse and we were lifted and hugged and loved and squeezed against a gorgeously comforting bosom. John used to hate it, pulling away, proper wee boy, but I loved it and showed it. Even when I was a man, going back off leave, and especially when embarkation leave was over, before walking down with Bill to York Street station, I lifted her up at the front door, smiled into her eyes, and kissed her wet cheek. On that woman upstairs in the bed the cheeks were like the insides of dried orange peel.

I gave Bill a dig and filled him full of importance. 'Come on,' I said, 'and I'll take you to McGrane's for a drink.'

We walked past spaces where houses and people had been blown away by German bombs, and where the lived-in houses all had paintwork that was dull and cracked.

At the top of Meadow Street somebody hailed me: 'Hugh, when did you get home?' As he hurried towards me up the steep hill, I didn't know him at first. He was tall, wearing an American checked shirt, Yankee navy dungarees, and stout yellow boots. Dock labourer was written all over him.

It came as a shock when I recognised Charlie Rusk, a schoolmate. Jaze, I thought, do I look as fixed and defined as that? We were both twenty-five, but it was the first time it came to me that twenty-five was such a bite into life. God, Charlie had permanent creases by his mouth and nose. Everybody who had been a boy with me was now well dug into manhood.

He gave me the smiling once over. 'What've you been doing with yourself, pulling the pud? You've dropped a couple of stone.'

I laughed, for the first time since I'd come home, really laughed. 'You're no Cary Grant yourself.'

'Where you heading?' He tried to make the question casual, but he wouldn't have been on the street at this time if there'd been a day's work at the docks.

'I'm heading for a wet. Coming?'

'Can't buy you one back.'

'So I'll get the bailiffs on you.'

He winked at Bill, who winked back, and we went through Jimmy McGrane's door smiling.

Inside, the cigarette-whiskey-porter mix and the soothing murmur of morning pub-talk did for me what the hush of the chapel does for the godly. A cheerful fire burned in the hearth, half a dozen customers sat contented over well-dressed pints. I led the way to a table in the corner near the fire and waited to catch Jimmy McGrane's eye. The publican was leaning on the counter, pointing something

18

out in the morning paper to two customers. Jimmy looked up and saw me, and at once came out from behind the counter and shuffled over on laceless shoes. I stood and he took my hand and shook it, as the other drinkers looked on in envy.

He was a bachelor of about sixty-five who had left a County Armagh farm at thirteen to serve his time to a skinflint publican on the Falls Road. He'd lived above the bar, in a loft, working a seventy-hour week, putting his money away. At fifty he'd bought his own bar with his own money, and now he had a nice steady house, well run, right on Spamount Street where the two sides met, where the clientele was fifty-fifty Catholic and Protestant, meeting as friends.

'Well, and welcome home, Hugh.'

'Nice to be home, Jimmy.'

White-haired, thin on top, Jimmy McGrane was the archetypal Irish publican, shrewd of eye, careful in his words. He smiled, nodded, looking appreciatively at my officer's gabardine, the wings, the two rings on my sleeves.

I pointed to Bill: 'This is our Bill. He's serving his time to the fitting in the yard. He should be at his work today, but he's taking a bottle of stout instead. A bottle and a half'n for Charlie Rusk, and the same for myself.'

'This one'll be my pleasure,' Jimmy said. Then he added: 'If I told you you were looking well, I'd be telling you a lie. You look as if you've had a hard oul war, Hugh.'

I was glad when he turned away to get the drinks. To a professor of crapulence like him, my face likely revealed my guzzling history, as clearly as the rings tell the age of a tree.

With the drinks before us, I relaxed with a long sigh. I raised my glass to Bill and Charlie, and inclined my head to Jimmy McGrane. 'Your good health.'

'You're safe home, now, Hugh,' Charlie said. And I felt it. It was good to be back. Good feelings began to rise in me again, I relaxed and we became company, the three of us. What I was feeling was true contentment. Bill was sipping, taking time over his stout, but Charlie and I saw our drinks off briskly. I was up at the counter ordering the next round when the door opened and John walked in.

'You couldn't wait, even at a time like this,' he said. 'Mother has just died.'

FOUR

———

I WAS SEVENTEEN WHEN Father died. So many things had happened since then that I'd forgotten what a working-class Belfast wake was like.

Already, for John and Bill, Aunt Nellie and all the other relations, the wake was the main thing. Mother had become notional, abstract. Her dying was the reason for this gathering, but, for this day and the next two, it was not Mother, but her waking that would matter. John and I were servants of the assemblies. We were putting in practice to greet all the visitors who would shortly be sorry for our trouble.

I had already been to the doctor and the undertaker and the man who wrote people off, the registrar of deaths on the

21

Donegall Road. All these miles had been covered thanks to a self-employed painter across the street, who had come to the door and, saying nothing, had handed me the keys of his Vauxhall.

Certainly, from Dad's wake I remembered the house packed with family connections – big families of big families on both sides – for two evenings. But since I'd been a non-drinker then I'd had no idea of the sheer quantity of the stuff that was on offer. In the early evening I was leaning against the china cabinet in the kitchen, resting, trying to get used to the idea that it was the done thing to knock it back, and laugh, and be cheerful, in the hours after Mother had died. Here in the kitchen, in the scullery, out in the hall, on the stairs, and even by the open door, uncles, cousins, relatives by marriage, friends and acquaintances were leaning, standing and sitting, drinking out of cups, mugs, glasses and straight from the bottle – branches and all, as the saying went – and three quarters of the women were sipping wine or sherry.

Mother's dying hadn't brought John and me any closer. We were communicating because we had to run the thing, but there was no easing of the distance between us; when he spoke to me it was to issue instructions.

This was all going to cost money. But John didn't have much, he told me. He seemed to think that I would understand why. I had paid out twenty-eight quid so far to Jimmy McGrane and it was clear that this wouldn't cover even half of the outlay. The insurance man had been – he was still out on the stairs, with a John Jameson in this hand – and had told us that Mother's policy would come to thirty pounds, which would pay for the funeral. It seemed fairly clear that I was expected to foot all other bills. Not that this worried me: I had come back from the war with plenty in the bank and my gratuity still to come when I was demobbed. Three years, two of them on officers' pay plus flying allowance, living mostly away from towns and drinking at mess prices, made for healthy savings.

I was tired. I stood with my eyes half closed. The women were talking to each other, in and out through each other. They sat on the sofa and on its arms, and on the chairs nearest to the fire. The whole house was full of their high chitter, with the men's talk providing the low notes in the background. How the women were able to communicate through the carrier wave of jabber was hard to work out, but they were getting through loud and clear, for every now and again a high-pitched laugh would escape the ground-returns as proof.

One of the undertaker's men appeared at the kitchen door. He was a small man, bald but for one long feather of white hair that lay across the pink shine of his head. I leaned towards him.

'Would you have a wee something?' he whispered. I had to put my ear to his mouth to hear him.

'Would a stout do, or something stronger?' I asked.

For reply he held his thumb and forefinger out – a half-glass of whiskey apart. I passed the request on through the crowd to the scullery and one of the uncles washed a cup and reached for the bottle.

By this time the women had seen the man at the door. They fell quiet. Then, with their eyes on the undertaker, the older women began to rock from side to side, and to make soft moaning noises. 'God look to our poor Betty,' Aunt Minnie said. 'Sowl, and He has her now,' Aunt Dolly put in, 'for if she's not in heaven the place is lying empty.'

All along the sofa and around the fire the sighing, the wails and the hand-wringing kept up. The man took the drink and nodded his thanks. He eased back into the crowd, and the moment he disappeared the babble broke out again, the lines of communication reopened, like criss-crossing radar beams. Once in a while a shrill scream of laughter would fly clear, reaching beyond the women by the fire to the hall outside, and into the parlour, where two strange men lifted and handled all that was left of my worn and wasted mother.

I was called to the front door. It was Billy Beattie, a man of about forty, a shipyard caulker from the next street, calling to pay his respects. 'Honest, Hugh, it seems no time at all since I was standing here at the door, at your father's wake.'

'It's eight years, Billy.'

'A decent man, Hugh, a decent respectable man. It was something awful, the way he went, and him only fifty-one.'

'Yes, and so it was, Billy. Would you like to come in for something?'

I stood back, called for Billy Beattie to be looked after, welcomed him past me, and stayed there in the early dark at the door in the lamplight. I wasn't sure about the way my father went, but when I had reached the age and time to think about it, I came to know how the news was brought.

It had been morning time and Mother was on her knees scrubbing the front step. Every now and then she would stop and brush the black hair away from her eyes with the back of her hand; her arms were guttered to the elbows with dirt. The street was almost empty and the sound of children chanting their multiplication tables came from the school at the corner. A few doors down, following a years-old

24

morning routine, the breadserver's horse had mounted the pavement and was standing at Maggie Pitcaithley's door, eating the heel of a loaf from Maggie's hand, his huge head reaching almost to the lintel of her door. Further down the street the herring man was calling. Everything was as it should have been – a typical morning scene. Mother wrung the floorcloth out until it reared in her hands like a grey snake, and then she dried the semi-circle of pavement in front of her doorstep. All up and down the street there were cleaned and scrubbed half-moons of pavement outside the other homes. Her hands were burning from the effects of the soap. She had risen from the floor, had gone into the scullery and was lathering her hands with the softer Lifebuoy soap when she heard a knock at the front door.

The knock was loud. It couldn't have been a neighbour; neighbours walked halfway up the hall and stopped and called softly: 'Are you in?' The knock came again, a double rap. She hurried out, wiping her hands on the rough sacking she used as an apron.

At the door stood a tall man, dressed in a narrow-trousered navy suit. He wore a high stiff collar and had a gold watch chain looped between his waistcoat pockets. He was about fifty years old; his face was long and narrow and he had ill-fitting false teeth. He peered at the sheet of paper he was holding, then at the number on the door. 'Are you Missus' – he looked again at the paper – 'Reilly?'

'That's right, sir.'

Mother called everyone in authority sir. In 1935, when the IRA were busy, I had been led home by the ear by our local cop, twenty minutes after ten o'clock curfew was up. I was fourteen and remember how humiliated I felt, hearing Mother plead: 'Sir, he's only a wee boy; he didn't know, sir.'

Mother was still wiping her hands, although they had dried long before.

'Can I come in?' The man spoke with the tone of authority and Mother stood back respectfully. To her dismay, he pushed past the parlour and went straight into the kitchen. At his feet were the bucket, the floorcloth, the scrubbing brush and the half-gallon-sized paint tin full of soft soap. She bent to clear them away, and had just dropped the brush and floorcloth into the empty bucket and straightened up when the man spoke again, this time sternly. 'Is that soap out of the shipyard?'

Indeed it was. Mixed with heavy engine oil, it was used to coat the slipways for a launch. It was customary for the workmen to scoop some of the soap into paint tins and carry it home. It was hard on the wives' hands, but it saved the price of Lifebuoy soap, and it did all right for rough scrubbing jobs.

'Was that soap lifted out of the yard?' he repeated.

'No, sir, no . . . well, it was, but it wasn't my man that gimme it, sir, it was a woman down the street.'

The man shook his head, exasperated, then, remembering, he held the piece of paper close to his eyes. 'You're Missus Reilly? Your husband's John Reilly?'

Mother's hands were almost tearing the sacking to shreds by now. 'He is, sir, but he didn't take that soap, so he didn't.'

Impatiently the man shook his head. 'I'm not talking about the soap, woman . . . ' His gaze shifted until it was fixed on a point some inches to one side of Mother's face. 'Your man's dead. There's been an accident. He fell off the staging on the Union-Castle boat.'

As Mother stared, the man turned and made for the door.

He stood awkwardly on the newly scrubbed step, waiting.

'They have him in the morgue,' he said, 'that's where he is ... Have you any boys?'

Mother answered him from the kitchen door. 'Yes, sir, I've three wee boys,' she said slowly.

The man took his watch out of his pocket, looked at it, pursed his lips, shook his head. 'It's usual to take a son on, when he's the age. But I don't know in this case. Still, we'll look at it, if you have one the age. Ask for Mister Magill, the manager.' And without looking back, he turned and walked across the street, to Duncairn Gardens and the tram back to the shipyard.

And Mother knew that the doubt in the man's voice over her son getting a job in the shipyard was because she herself was a Half-and-Half. Her father was Catholic, her mother Protestant. The girls were brought up in the mother's faith and the boys in the father's, so she had three Catholic brothers. Since Dad was a complete, entire Protestant, that made me and John and Bill quadroons, masquerading as Protestants, but anyway, that's how Mother learned about Dad's death, so I just nodded to Billy Beattie when he said that he was sorry.

At the time a story was going around that Dad didn't fall, but was pushed, because of Mother. I was told this when I was fifteen by a playmate whose father was an Orangeman and an iron turner in the yard. It didn't worry me now, anyway, the war just over had killed whatever little interest I'd ever had in the religious war.

I went back to where Uncle Alec was sitting on one stair, with Uncle Sammy and John on a stair above. They were Mother's brothers. Like her, they were small and dark and quick in their movements. Both had served in the trenches in the First War. Sometimes, before our war, they had begun to talk about their experiences, but had run into the indifference of each new generation to past history, but now John was happy to swap experiences with both.

'Of course, you fellows had lorries to carry you about – we had to march nearly everywhere,' Uncle Alec said, after a long suck at the neck of a bottle of stout.

'There was still plenty of soldiering,' John said. 'I spent any amount of time lying in holes in the ground in France and Holland.'

'You should have played it clever and joined the air force, like Hughie,' Uncle Sammy said, with a wink at me. 'You didn't catch them lying in holes in the ground.'

Uh oh.

I was waiting for it and it came: 'I couldn't for the bladdy life of me have spent the war in the air force,' John said, in his deepened voice and English accent. 'All that Brylcreem and aftershave. A bigger bunch of fruit merchants I've never seen. A day in the army would have killed them.'

Uncle Sammy was full of fun and generous in his nature. I could see the dismay on his face. Before the sharp anger took hold of me I jumped the stairs to the bottom and pushed into the kitchen.

'Hello there, handsome!'

I turned and the white rage ebbed away. It was Alma, my cousin, Alma Conway, Uncle Sammy's daughter, my full cousin. She'd just thrown her coat over the back of the sofa and was standing half a foot away from me, dark hair, full lips, plenty, but not too much of her. I put my arms out and she came to me, and the way we kissed silenced every woman in the room.

'Now now, that'll do.' The women were rolling their eyes, as I held her out and admired her, my hands slow to leave her waist.

Aunt Sal, Alma's mother said: 'You're too near in the blood.'

I remembered that Catholics were almost in terror of cousins making it together.

'Come you here and sit by me,' Aunt Sal scolded, somehow making room for Alma beside her, but when she sat down I went and hunkered down at her knees.

'You're looking smashing,' I told her, 'I suppose you're married now.' I was wondering what would happen if I were to lift the hem of her skirt and edge it back beyond what our navigators called the PLE – the prudent limit of endurance.

Her legs were stained brown. Her knees looked sunburnt and gorgeous. As the women held their breath I looked up into her brown eyes. Alma was acknowledging my signal.

'No, I'm not married yet,' she smiled.

I took her hands. 'I'll be best man, since I'm too near in the blood,' I said.

The women laughed, I kissed Aunt Sal and went into the scullery to get drinks for the newcomers. I poured sherry into two eggcups and then I stood for a moment with my eyes closed. When I opened them Alma was there.

'You look done in, Hugh.'

'I'm knackered. Yesterday I was in Italy.'

A curtain separated the scullery from the kitchen. I suddenly kissed Alma and in the three seconds that it lasted I had my guess confirmed.

'You're awful,' she whispered.

'I'll give you awful,' I said, and went into the kitchen,

gave out the drinks, and then stood at the door, looking out into the gaslit January night.

From somewhere in the harbour came the distinctive, doleful sound of a Kelly's coal boat making ready to sail. Out in Duncairn Gardens a tram slowly ground past; a sudden blue flash behind the roofs of the houses opposite gave me a fix on its position. From the Spencer Basin came the shrill whoop of a warship's siren. The tide was on the move: the berthing masters were busy.

Leaving Belfast three years before, I'd leant over the rail of the Heysham boat, watching the outline of the Antrim hills above the lough's rim, black against the sky. Beside me a sergeant navigator, who had travelled home with me two weeks earlier, had said: 'I suppose you're wondering, like me, if we'll ever see this again.'

'Well, I suppose, indirectly, I was,' I told him. 'What I was really thinking was that it's not much, but Christ help us, it's all we've got.'

The navigator's name was Pollock and he came from Larne. He was somewhere in Romania now for good, his Wimpey making a big hole in the ground. He was one of the fruit merchants that John had mentioned on the stairs a while back.

Somebody was beside me. 'Terrible time to come home, Hugh,' Uncle Sammy said. 'But at least you're home, that's the best part.'

I didn't answer.

After a minute he said: 'You know, Hugh, it was the same after the last war.' He searched for the words. 'We were all strung up, too.' He laughed. 'I can mind a real murdering match broke out at Osborne Street corner. It was at a pitch-and-toss school. The men were just out of the army, back from France, all out of work. The game ended up with split heads, busted noses, fat lips. Know what it was over? The fellow doing the tossing was spotted with rosary beads wrapped round his tossing hand. He had headed the pennies five times. They reckoned he was cheating.'

I laughed and went back inside.

FIVE

T HE AIR WAS THICK with the smell of drink and
cigarette smoke, but not dense enough to smother the
sweetish scent of the wreaths and the new-varnished coffin.
The noise was louder than ever. The parlour door was open
a little and I peeped in. The undertaker's men were tidying
the curtains by the window behind the coffin. One of them
nodded me in: 'Would you like to see her?'

She was dressed to the neck in some sort of shiny, satiny
garment. They had Max Factored the grey that had been
there in her face when she was dying, to a warmer look, and
under the veil the outlines were softened. This was why
people said that the dead were at peace; it was because

undertakers made them look as if they were. If Mother had been left as she was at the moment of her dying, peace wouldn't have been the word that came to mind.

Her hair hadn't looked right on her deathbed and it didn't look any more natural now, pulled back tightly, like a school-teacher's. I pulled the veil back, and as the two men clicked their tongues I put my hand under her head, lifted it, and fluffed her hair forward, loosening it up. Then I laid her head back on the pillow and replaced the veil.

The men put on their coats and went out and the mourn-ers began to come in. The women were well able to handle it, the more that they were the ones who did the crying.

'She's just lovely.'

'Ah well, she's at peace, God take care of her.'

'There'll be no more suffering there now for her, Nellie.'

The men could only stare and shift their feet.

'Well, she got away, anyway.'

'Aye, she was a good woman.'

'You'll miss her, boys.'

At this, Bill began to cry, turning away after one sight of the corpse. I went to him, put an arm around him. With his face against my chest he shook and sobbed. I didn't know what to say to him, except, 'I know, I know, kid.' I felt a hand on my shoulder. It was Alma. She took over, holding Bill close.

In releasing Bill, I rested my hand on her waist, dropped it to her hip, before leaving go. When her back was to me I saw the cream of her neck, the round hips. A black line, a simulated stocking seam, had been ruled up the back of her well-formed legs. Under the thin material of her blouse her bra straps could be seen. There was no bulge below them.

Beyond Alma was the coffin head and Mother's made-up face, more indistinct at this distance, more unreal. I pushed through the mourners. My mind was running rough, like an engine with a mag drop. I went into the scullery and poured a whiskey.

'You're changed away beyond description. You're looking what you might call interesting,' said Jean Midgley, a childless, breasty married woman of twenty-eight, who lived in Adam Street. I knew her age because she'd been in John's class at school.

John was back from the parlour. 'For God's sake he's light enough in the head without telling him that kind of stuff. Sure he spends most of his time looking at himself in the glass,' he said. The drink, and the long day, were telling on him as well. His face was flushed and his eyes were red. I had a three-inch advantage in height over him, but he looked all right – certainly more compact than I was. He had good shoulders and was well muscled. There was no reason why he shouldn't fancy himself with Jean Midgley. Her husband was in the navy and she had a lively eye for the men if her opening move to me was anything to go by.

'Well, Hugh has plenty to look at in the glass. There's any number would run away with him.' This came from Aunt Minnie, with a murmur of agreement from Jean Midgley.

'Don't you be taking too much drink, boy, you've all these people to run home, you know.' John's voice tore into my nerves like the first bite of a circular saw into green wood.

'Didn't they teach you to frigging drive in the army, sergeant?' I was standing beside him, deliberately coming the officer. As usual, he was stuck for the quick word. I went out into the hall and stood with my back against the coats, shaking my head.

Before the war he had frigged me about from arsehole to breakfast time. I used to read a book a day from the library; I read as I walked and talked and ate and it used to get right up his jacksie: 'Why don't you go out and play like the other kids? Why are you always hanging around the house like a jinny wing?' He was top man in the house, so I'd had to swallow it.

Often I was literally kicked out into the street. And when I got there I would go and find my mates, and lead them in a wild escapade, scaling one Everest after another, just to show John that I was no jinny wing.

Once, I'd climbed the ivy-covered trellis in front of the local Presbyterian church, and hidden from sight behind the leaves, I took out my tiny dick, squeezed its top to get a fine spray effect, and peed over a group of churchgoers, just entering the porch. They looked up, and one of them, his hair blowing in the wind, put his hand out. 'There's a wee touch of rain about this morning, Agnes,' he said, and my mate and I nearly fell out of the ivy laughing.

John had a three-year lead on me. At, say, nineteen over sixteen, that's a hell of a distance. Now, I was twenty-five to his twenty-eight, and I had fighting form that John knew nothing about. I wasn't about to be kicked out any more.

Bill came out to the hall and stood beside me. 'This is drastic.' It was one of his favourite words. 'They do nothing but laugh and cha ha. Are all wakes like this?'

'All of ours are.' It occurred to me as I said it that maybe Protestant wakes were not like this at all: more likely, ours reflected the Catholic influence in the family. 'They think she wouldn't like too much crying.'

'Well, I can't get used to it. Christ, where do they put the stuff? I tried drinking stout with you this morning and you can keep it.'

I laughed. 'The first drink I ever had was in an English pub. That day I sank six of them. I wish that first one had made me spew.'

'Don't be daft. Tommy Lyle said he travelled over with you in the Heysham boat and you'd a head like a rock.'

'The one thing I've learned out of this war is that nobody has a head like a rock for drink. If it doesn't get you the day you take it, it'll get you later, and the more you take, the more you'll suffer.'

'I suppose you had to watch yourself in the officers' mess, anyway.'

'Well, yes, but I managed not to watch myself a good few times. Just as an example, after listening to a group captain from the south of Ireland running down northern Protestants, I told him his arse was out of the porthole. He then told me that he was a Protestant himself and I told him that, in that case, his arse and balls and all were out of the porthole.'

'That's not your form. You were never very Orange.'

'I'm still not, but I wasn't having any Free-Stater telling me the score.'

'What happened?'

'The usual – everybody clearing their throats and a change of subject.'

'Talking about officers, did you know that John failed a commission in the army?'

I nodded. That was another thing.

Just before I flew out to North Africa I'd been summoned to the office of the CO of the ferry unit at Portreath in Cornwall. We were ready to go off next morning.

'I say, flight sergeant, would you call into the orderly room and fill in commissioning papers? There's a good chap.'

I filled the papers in and duly flew off. When I got to the transit camp at Almaza near Cairo it was to find that a board had been arranged for a few days ahead. I attended the board and had a chat about the trials and troubles of being a pilot. It was clear that I'd passed the thing but I'd said nothing to Mother.

In the bloody meantime, John had written home to announce that he was going up for second lieutenant. In the same week the word came through to Mother that I had passed and John had failed. She found out about my promotion for the first time when the air force asked her to return the order book for the few bob a day allotment that I was making to her: 'Henceforth provision for you must be made through Messrs Cox and King's Bank, London, since your son has been granted a commission in the rank of Pilot Officer.'

I collapsed on the stairs beside Uncle Sammy and closed my eyes.

'Why don't you turn in?' he said.

'I wish I could, but somebody has to drive the visitors home.'

He looked closely at me. 'Are you OK for driving?'

'Oh, I'll take it easy. But I hope it won't be long.' I wasn't hurting his feelings saying that – Uncle Sammy just lived along by Carrick Hill, maybe fifteen minutes' walk at the most.

Just then the crowd made way for a new visitor, a girl with a small suitcase in her hand. She came up the hall and, to my surprise, stopped when she came opposite to me. She was small, about twenty-two, with fair hair down to her collar, then turned up, in the fashion. Nice-looking, but not exciting. Since she was looking at me and smiling and saying nothing, I stood up.

'You must be Hugh.'

I stepped down to the hall beside her.

She stood on her toes and kissed my cheek. 'I'm Annie.'

'Annie?' I was puzzled to hell's gates.

'You know, Annie Longley, from Bangor.'

Suddenly John was in the hall. He wrapped his arms around her and they kissed. A good one, too. Then he led her into the kitchen.

'Who the hell's that?' I muttered to Bill.

'That's Annie Longley. She's engaged to John.'

I remembered something about a girlfriend in a letter from home. 'Engaged? Christ!'

'By post. A couple of months ago.'

The letters from Mother had stopped about then.

'Well good luck to her if she can make it with that dry bread.'

I was making a face after finishing another whiskey when I heard my name being called. In the kitchen Annie Longley was sitting near the fire, warming her hands. With her coat off she looked pretty, in a woollen dress, green, with black doodahs. 'C'mere you, Hugh, I want to take a look at you,' she said.

When a new woman joins a family she joins it good, I thought. She was talking to me as if she was my sister. I smiled nicely at her. 'How do you do? You took me by surprise, I'm afraid.'

'God,' Annie glanced at Alma, the nearest one to her in age, 'would you look at him! Tall, dark and starving. I say,

38

Alma, who's going to be busy with the girls? I'm pleased to meet you.'

'In that case, I'm pleased to meet you, too.'

'Have you a girl, yet?'

All that was missing was the dimple. She had an easy confidence. I was betting she was bossy, really. I pointed to Alma. 'I fancy her, but they won't let me.'

Alma was carrying it off well, with a laugh that went with the crowd's.

'Anyway,' I went on, falling in with the banter, 'I haven't had time to look around me. I only just got here this morning.' I ran a hand through my hair. 'Seems like a month ago.'

'Well, although it's a sad time, it's nice to see you, I've met the man now, after all I've been hearing.'

'I didn't know you two were engaged.'

John broke in: 'You're supposed to offer congratulations, or didn't you know?' He was well away; his focusing was up the chute.

I smiled. 'I'm very happy for you.'

She inclined her head. The listening women nodded and smiled too.

'What you see before you, Annie, is Belfast's answer to Gregory Peck. What do you think of the wavy hair? They're not allowed into the air force without it,' John said.

This time there was no chance of handling the tightness in my chest. This time, I'd had John. 'And what you have there with his arm round you,' I said, 'is somebody who's been asking for a busted lip since I arrived here this morning.' My voice was low, I was smiling; I had straightened up and my legs were spread; my jaw was tightened against the risk of dislocation; I drew in a lungful of air, and let a quarter out.

'What did you just say to me?' John's hand came away from Annie's shoulder; his brow came down. 'What did you say?'

'Here's what I said: you've been asking for a busted lip since I came in here this morning. Here's more: you've been treating me like shit all day. And here's more still: I can take you. OK?'

'Sweet Jesus!' Uncle Sammy moved in between us. 'Boys, boys, what's this?'

John was on his feet, shrugging off Annie's hold. 'Right, outside, you.'

All around the room there was a scuffling of feet and scraping of chairs as the women scrambled to get out of the way. Uncle Alec grabbed my arm. I didn't resist, I just smiled into John's face, needling him into action. Inside my head there was a high-frequency oscillator. I was pushed back, as John gave way to pressure from Uncle Sammy.

'Now, lads, this is terrible altogether.'

The women froze. I caught sight of Bill, pale, riveted; near him, Alma Conway was wide-eyed, watching.

'Why don't you shake and forget it?' The suggestion came from a younger man, somebody's son-in-law. 'Your mother's in her coffin.'

'You'll be sorry in the morning, Hugh,' a neighbour man said.

John was staring at me, puzzled, resentful. Suddenly he lifted his open hand and swung it. The blow caught the top of my head as I rolled away.

One question had been answered: John knew nothing about fighting. He was off-balance, his eyes were full of fury, so they weren't watching, and his head was there for the hitting. I turned it with a transparent feint and let him have it with a short left.

His eyes glazed as he started to go down, but he cannoned into Uncle Sammy and that kept him on his feet. As the women screamed and the men shouted, John threw himself at me, wrapping his arms around my waist; I was wrestled into the hall. I grabbed a handful of crotch and as he bent over and let me go I caught him with an uppercut that sent him backwards into the parlour. Before he could gather himself, I followed up, hit him again, and this time he fell crashing into the china cabinet. The cover shattered and the contents were showered with glass fragments.

The others had stopped at the parlour door in horror. As John went finally to his knees, face-down on the floor, I stepped back, licking my fist. Some projection caught me, rib-high; I half turned; the coffin had been jolted almost off its trestles. I turned the whole way, and found myself looking down into it.

Heaving and gasping, and finally sobbing, I left John lying on the floor, flung myself past the crowd at the door, and ran into the street.

It was raining. Bareheaded, coatless, I ran, blind from the rain and the tears, and in my head, two images were clear, distinct and defined, although wildness churned and boiled and seethed all around them. One was the dead, still face of my mother, disturbed in her coffin, the hair that I had loosened fallen over one eye. The other was John's face: throughout the whole fight, all the way from the first slap to the final punch, his face had been unguarded, and in his eyes, at the end, just before he went down, there was only perplexity and helplessness.

SIX

T HE YOUNG AVIATOR lay dying,
    And as in the hangar he lay, he lay,
To the fitters who round him were standing
These last parting words he did say;

Take the cylinders out of my kidneys,
The connecting rod out of my brain, my brain,
From the small of my back take the camshaft,
And assemble the engine again.

That's a Royal Flying Corps song, that, Ginger. Oh, what
nice eyes you've got, Ginger. Nice thighs you've got,
Ginger.

Best of order there. What's your name, oul son? Dan what?
Dan Byrne? Well the best of order Dan Byrne, till I sing a
wee song:

> Now the foreman said to me
> When I came in rather late,
> As he grabbed me by the bollocks
> And he threw me through the gate,
> If you can't come fucking early
> Then you can't come fucking late,
> When you're working down the sewer
>   shovelling shit.
>
> When you're working down the sewer,
>   shovelling up manure,
> That's where the navvy does his bit, shovelling shit.
> You can hear the shovels ring, with a ting a ling a ling
> When you're working down the sewer
>   shovelling shit.

OK, Ginger, OK, I'm going. In a wee minute.

Where's my coat?

Alla best, Dan Byrne, alla best, Dicky, alla best, all.

Here's one more song. One more:

> In Dublin's fair city, I searched for her diddy,
> But I'm frigged if I found one on Molly Malone.
> With her chest flat and narrow, she wheels her
>   wheelbarrow
> For that's all she's fit for, poor Molly Malone.

43

I'm an orphan, Ginger. I'm a member of the Protestant Orphan Society. Did I tell you, Ginger?

I'll get this taxi. I've got lira. Jesus God, but I'm tired . . .

SEVEN

WHATEVER HAD LED UP to this latest piss-up, I was in a real bed, at least.

I'd woken up in some places, I'll say. Once, I'd come to my senses in a bakery in Naples, up a needle-narrow side street, lying on top of a pile of two hundredweight flour bags. Did my uniform the world of good, that did. Then what about the time I'd crashed eight feet through an open grating in the street in Tunis, right on top of a Yankee poker school. Medical orderlies they were; I'd landed in a sick quarters, woke up with that iodine-looking stuff on my bruises and abrasions. Now at least I was in a proper bed, and it was a Belfast bed. Some woman was saying good morning to me, speaking Belfast.

I kept my eyes tight shut.

The world outside this warm, cosy bed could get stuffed. There was no such thing as a good morning.

I closed my hand around the breast I'd woken up holding, and squashed up to the hips that were so obligingly close. This was much better. The bad feelings that had just shoved the tips of their noses into my business were edged out by better urges. My left hand slid under and took the other breast.

I was now ready for forgetsies. The instrument hadn't yet been made that could measure my readiness. I could have driven it between two courses of brick.

First, the works. Then back to sleep until, oh, let's say . . . 1999. No, let's not bother waking up at all . . .

With faint irritation I felt a movement. Her head was turning. I felt a soft cheek against mine, then the woman turned to face me and my hands were dispossessed of diddies. As well as that I had lost all the nice, hippy comfort. But my left arm didn't go to waste on the waist. It pulled her close, as two arms came around my neck. My right arm knew what to do in this situation, and my dry lips were suddenly being kissed.

'Good morning.'

I closed my eyes even more tightly. Civility is superfluous when death looks a bargain.

I rolled on top, receiving expert help halfway. I took the weight on my forearms, laid my head alongside hers, who-ever she was, and prayed that the climax to which I had committed myself would burst a blood vessel, finish me with a stroke, or at least leave me a vegetable.

I began slowly, then worked up to a pounding, driving rhythm. I wanted my heart to explode and my blood pressure to split veins and arteries. Failing this, I would have settled for blindness, deafness and paralysis. I sought and quickly found purchase for my toes at the bed end, and with the next thrust, drove the woman up on her pillow, but soon we were rearing and plunging, rising and falling together. She was crying; no, the cries were coming from two people, and that was surprising, until I found that I was helping. I was irritated, where there was room in the red whirl for irritation, by the woman's response: this wasn't her suicide attempt, it was mine. Still, I put my lips on hers and found that her jaw was set, fixed, by one frenzied, prolonged orgasm, but I kept the kiss there because my own was coming and it took so long, was so fierce and so bitter and wild that it seemed as if all my wishes had been granted and I was dying of the Indian burn.

When it was all drained, I rolled until we were facing each other. My eyes opened and it came to me that, although I would rest, there'd be no sleep now.

I felt her finger on my cheek, tracing the course of my tears. 'I know,' she said, 'I know, Hughie.'

For the first time, I looked at her. I sat up, shaking my head. I rolled sideways out of bed and stood up, bare, ball naked. I squinted at her.

She looked good, dressed in nothing but a sheet, and she wasn't one of those women who pull the sheet up to their chin when a man is looking, because the folds ended just below her full, spread breasts. Her hair was deep auburn and she had the clear, clean skin that goes with it. Her colour was high, and no wonder, since we'd just taken Olympic gold, the two of us. I looked down on her and she smiled back, and the curves that I knew all about were moulding the sheet into some sheet, by Christ.

47

'I know you,' I said. I had to have another try at the words before it came out right, and she laughed. Her voice was warm and deep and it made me smile a little, and sit on the edge of the bed. Her eyes were very blue. I wondered about this in a redhead. 'I know you,' I said.

'Christ, you ought to.'

'Why? Why should I know you?'

'One, I rescued you last night from whatever it was that you wanted to do – probably lie on the road and get run over by a bus – and two, I was in the class below you at school.'

My brain, like my mouth, was packed with plaster of Paris. I smacked my tongue, 'Is there a cup of rosy?'

She climbed out of bed, grabbed a bathrobe from behind the door, stepped into slippers. 'Yes, I'll get you a drop,' she said. I followed her downstairs.

I was in a typical two-up, two-down kitchen stroke living room. It was well furnished by kitchen-house standards, indeed, sumptuously so, moneylender level, as we used to say, with decent quality carpet on the floor, a comfortable settee, an easy chair, three well-made upright chairs, a heavy oak table, curtains that matched the carpet and suite, and crystal and brass all over the place. In bare feet it was cosy and that was rare in this belt of Belfast.

Still without a stitch on, I flopped down on to the settee and sighed, and the sigh came from the dead centre of my heart. I jumped up, went after the woman into a de luxe scullery. She'd had the place done over. It was twice the size of the average scullery. There'd been pushing done out to the yard, and covering done with beaverboard and a felt roof. There were neat, tidy cupboards, a shining new sink, and a ritzy-looking cooker. This was what my mother would have called a babby house, a honeymoon house.

The tea was drawing, the cups were china, with matching milk jug, all placed on a mahogany veneer tray.

'Want any chow?' I noted the Americanism. She was looking over her shoulder and, even in a bathrobe, she looked dressy, with shoulders straight, chin up, and shining, chestnut hair that just exactly covered the back of her neck.

I wanted to touch her, but I didn't; I carried the tray in and sat on the settee, holding it, as she poured the tea. She took the tray and, pulling a table from a nest, she set the tray on it. 'Don't burn yourself,' she joked, glancing at my bare, crossed legs. She crossed hers and her robe fell open. I looked down, after one eyeful.

'For the present I don't want to hear about last night,' I said, when the tea had done its work. 'I can't think why you've been so kind to me, but save that up, too. Just tell me why I know your face.'

She was looking down at her cup, stirring her tea. 'I'm called Mary Waugh.' She gave me a quick glance; defensive.

Some memory faintly tugged, one that contradicted the carpet and curtains and, indeed, all of her poise and confidence. We always remember the schoolmates in our class and above us, but hardly ever the ones below us. There was something about her, though.

'I'm the one who was fed by the teachers,' she said, looking full at me now, watching my reaction.

Then it came. In times when none of us at school had anything more than the bare subsistence; when over half the kids in the class were unable, on a Monday morning, to hand in the penny that was needed for coal to warm the classroom, poor Mary Waugh had trailed the rest of us by a distance.

Orphaned when she was eleven, an aunt had taken Mary into her house in Brougham Street, but all that Mary got was houseroom. The girl slept on an old mattress on the floor and was fed by neighbours, while the aunt babbled to herself in drink, and begged and sold herself to buy more drink.

Through it all Mary had been a solitary child. She had kept herself as neat as her cast-offs allowed, the teachers gave her raw egg and milk beaten up in a cup in the mornings, and sent out for soda bread for her to butter and eat at lunch times. That was all I could recall.

Oh, yes, there was something else, something I'd heard on one of my leaves home, part of the talk at the corner of the street of an evening: Mary Waugh had gone on the game. It hadn't surprised me, nor had it shocked me. What the hell about it? Sure we all pissed in the open yard and only used the closet for the other. Who wanted to lay down standards?

I gulped tea down and took a more informed inventory. Certainly the place looked like the home of a cracking good whore.

'I know you now,' I said.

She laughed. 'And I know you, Reilly. When you were at school you just didn't give a goddam, did you?'

Chow. And goddam. The Yanks are coming, the Yanks are coming.

'You were a cheeky bastard with brains,' she said. 'Christ, I loved you to smithereens, the way you stood up to the teachers.'

It was nice to be taken out of the present, but this was 1946, time to catch up. I was ready now.

'You're a gorgeous woman grown, and you certainly looked after me last night. I can remember only singing and odd bits. Did I call you Ginger?'

She nodded, with mock disgust.

'How did we meet?'

'You ran past me on York Street, as I was getting out of a car. You were wild-looking, no coat or hat, crying, shaking your head. I watched and you ran into Mulgrew's pub at the corner of Trafalgar Street. I ran in after you and everybody thought I was with you, including yourself. You and Dicky Walters sang air force songs and knocked shots of whiskey back. You took a liking to some guy in the snug, some docker, and you and Dicky filled him full of whiskey as well. As usual, when you'd spent pounds and couldn't drink any more, Mulgrew gave you the bum's rush.'

Bum's rush and shots of whiskey. I was getting to like Mary Waugh. She was like Lend Lease aid at a time of need.

'Dicky Walters? Was he there? Last I heard of him he was captured by the Japs.'

'So he was, and he's home with three years' pay, throwing it round him like he'd won the Irish Sweep.'

Like the song about O'Riley's daughter, suddenly a thought came into my head. 'Would you put me up for a bit, Mary? I'll pay you top whack.' Another thought: 'You're not fixed up with a man or anything?'

Mary put her cup down and the laughing took her so suddenly that she had to put the back of her hand over her mouth. 'In a way of speaking you could say that I'm fixed up.' She eyed me sideways. 'Do you know what I'm talking about?'

'Are you on the game?' I sat waiting for her answer as if I'd asked her if she worked in York Street mill.

'That's right.' Her manner was cool; she sat, waiting.

'Does that mean that I can't stay here?'

'No.'

'OK,' I stood up, stretched. The clock said nine in the morning. 'I want to take a bath, then breakfast. What do you do for a bath?' Usually it was the zinc job, hanging in the yard.

'Follow me,' said Mary, and led me upstairs to surprise number umpteen: the small back bedroom was a bathroom, done in soft green, and for heaven's sake there was a shower, properly plumbed. She'd had a good war. But then she'd fought a hard enough one before any of us had even heard of Hitler.

I let the shower run cold. The brain started to work as I stood gasping and goose-pimpling. I had no clothes to wear; what I had were in a sorry pile on the bedroom floor. And contact would have to be made with Bill. And I could have done with a drink. I let the water drum on my scalp and stood until a fit of trembling told me to leave it.

In the bedroom, as I towelled myself pink, Mary was tying up her hair.

'Dicky Walters can go and pick up whatever clothes you need. I'll wash those.'

I stared. She'd been reading my mind. 'But how do we get in touch with Dicky?'

'I told him last night to call here this morning. I hope he'll remember.'

I pulled on my damp trousers, deciding to ditch the underpants. 'I have a query for you,' I said.

'Oh, yes?'

'How do you like the way I'm keeping the courtesies between us since we got out of bed?'

'Are you finding it hard?'

'Oh, but yes.'

'Well, then I like it.'

A knock came to the door and Mary went to open it. I went down to the kitchen and stopped in astonishment. Dicky Walters was sitting on one of the easy chairs, nearly lost in its depth. There'd never been much of him, but this guy was almost unrecognisable. His face was gaunt and his chest was chicken.

'Jesus Christ,' I said, 'you look like a doorman in a knocking shop – hard ridden.'

I hadn't seen him since back in forty-one. At that time he was an air-gunner. It was just after gunners had been raised to sergeant and officer rank, and I, at that time a leading aircraftman, was impressed by Dicky's stripes and his flying record.

His stripes were gone; he was a plain-nothing ranker. He saw my eyes on his sleeves and on his chest where the flying brevet should have been. He gave a nervous snicker. 'Sure I told you all about it in Mulgrew's last night.'

Before the war he'd had a Fred Astaire smile, loose and friendly; now, well, his mouth hung more or less permanently open, his lips slack. He fidgeted and moved all the time, and there were tiny twitches and tremors near his eyes. I knew the eye signs: certain flying operations brought those on, but Dicky was in the worst overall shape I'd ever seen for a serving airman.

The snicker came again. 'It was the old LMF.' He meant Lack of Moral Fibre, air-forcese for cowardice. 'They busted me down to AC2.'

'How many operations did you do?'

'Thirty-one. The tour was forty. In Blenheims. In daylight.'

I shook my head in disbelief. More than half of the Blenheim crews that flew in daylight at the start of the war were shot down. 'What kind of job did they give you?' I asked.

'What do you think – the latrines.'

Jesus, I thought. An officer pilot in our squadron, after half a dozen trips over Balkan and Italian targets, saw one night what an Me 110 night-fighter did to two of his squadron kites. That was the last we saw of him. But instead of being reduced to the ranks and put on shithouse fatigues, he was transferred to Air-Sea Rescue on Walrus amphibians. One rule for officers, another for the men.

Dicky was pulling at a cigarette so hard that brown streaks had appeared along the paper.

'I suppose the fuckpots sent you out to the Far East as well,' I said.

He gave his whinnying laugh. 'Bloody sure they didn't. I was having such a bad time of it – they were crucifying me, on the station where I'd flown as a flight sergeant – that I volunteered for overseas. I'll tell you one thing, Hughie, it was a frigging sight better under the Japs in Singapore than it was in England. At least as POWs we were all the same. The only thing was the grub. There was none.'

'Where did you sleep last night?'

'Well I wasn't as lucky as you,' his eyes went to Mary, in her bathrobe beside me. 'I stayed in Carrick House, the corporation doss house, where all the nobs hang out.'

'I'm staying here, pro tem.'

'Jammy bastard.'

'I need clothes, look at me.' He did, and I took a long one at him, and my shake, no matter how bad, was never in his league. 'Could you call at our house, see our Bill, and organise some clothes from my kit?'

'Sure. And Hughie . . .'

'Yeah?'

'While you're sorting yourself out, could I knock about with you?'

I felt Mary's hand on my arm, squeezing gently. 'Dicky, didn't you look after me last night?'

'Well, you were in a hell of a state, you know.'

'So. You and I are mates, OK? Hurry up and do that job. I'll be stuck here, forced to stay with Mary Waugh till you rescue me.'

His face all smiles, he gave me a stage wink and went.

'And you think you've got trouble?' Mary said. 'He's been kicked out of the house. His old fellow's disowned him, ever since he lost his stripes.'

'Well, as a matter of fact, I do think I've got trouble.' I went all gloomy again, but I was following Mary Waugh up the stairs even as I gloomed.

EIGHT

MARY'S HOUSE WAS IN the middle of Lewis Street, only five minutes' walk from my own. Twenty minutes after Dicky Walters had left he was back with Bill and a suitcase full of clothes. In the bijou splendour of her home, Bill was almost struck dumb in the presence of Mary Waugh. She had come downstairs in a blue dress, high at the shoulders, and shaped just loosely enough under her bosom to show what she had without being vulgar about it. Her hair was brushed smooth and she was wearing the sort of nylons I'd only ever seen before when I was training in Canada and the USA. When she sat down to meet Bill she was showing only half an inch above the knees, but he seemed almost in distress with the effort of trying to look away from them.

'I suppose you know one another,' I said.

'Hello, Bill.' He'd been blushing since she'd appeared, so he couldn't go any redder. 'I've some messages to do,' she said. 'I'll be back for lunch and you're welcome to stay and have something with Hugh.'

'It's OK,' I said. 'We'll get something out, but if you want us we'll be down in the Greenmount.

Before leaving, Mary touched Bill on the sleeve: 'I'm very sorry about your mother. She was a lovely, friendly woman and she always had a word for me.'

Bill smiled and nodded and gave a little shift of the shoulders as she left. When the door closed behind her, he closed his eyes and swallowed.

Down in the Greenmount I ordered a pint. My nerves felt exposed for inches of their length. We sat, the three of us, by the window. The sound of riveting from the shipyard rolled like a distant firefight across the basin. Behind it, from Short's, was the noise of an aircraft engine on its test-bed being run up to maximum revs, and held. When I'd been away I hadn't remembered these sounds of home.

'John has a hell of a peeper,' Dicky Walters said. 'A real wheeker.'

I looked at Bill. 'What's the temperature at home?'

'After the fight the women tidied things up and the old-timers knocked the whiskey back and talked about what it was like after the First War. They were saying it's nerves.'

'Now, on top of everything else, you're batchy,' Dicky said.

'I didn't know you could fight like that,' Bill was blowing out his cheeks. 'My God, you're mustard.'

'For Jaze' sake, I could bate him with my cap,' Dicky was regarding me in a warm, matey way.

'What's on the programme now?' Bill asked.

'I'm staying with Mary Waugh.' Saying it gave me a tingle; for all the trouble I was in, waking up in the morning could have been a hell of a lot worse.

Bill glanced at Dicky, then at me. 'Um . . . there's something you don't know there.'

'You mean she's a brass nail?'

He looked blank.

'On the game,' I explained.

Bill was gaping. He looked to be only in his depth by a millimetre. 'Everybody round here knows her,' he said.

'Wait'll I tell you,' Dicky said. 'She's high class. High American officers she goes with, and nobody else. Nobody.' He turned to Bill. 'I near died when she came into Mulgrew's with Hugh here. Mary usually wouldn't go near it. She saw me, got me to bring Hugh into the snug, then she stayed with him till he more or less fell off his feet.' He laughed, coming back to me. 'There was another guy in there, a nice guy, a docker. He gave Mary and me a hand to get you out into the taxi. Before that, we knocked him full, between the two of us. Nice fellow, he was.'

Bill sat drinking his orange juice. 'Look Hugh, it's not me. I like her. But it's just more ammunition for Lord Bunkum, with his stupid accent.'

'He's all right,' I frowned at him. 'I'm the one that wrecked the house, you know. He was just badgering, but I was the wrecker.'

Bill sighed. 'Are you not coming home again?'

'You stay and stick up for me.' I gave him a wink.

Soon after, Mary came in. 'What's the word on the

funeral?' she asked Bill.

'Ten in the morning.'

She saw me making a face. 'You're going, aren't you?'

'Oh aye, but I'm not looking forward to it.'

Mary looked at me and smiled. 'I knew you'd be there. Whatever you're going to do, do it before tea time. It'll take the whole evening to get your clothes ready.'

If the funeral was set for ten o'clock, then the service in the parlour would be ten minutes earlier. I set off from Mary's at a quarter to. She walked with me as far as the corner of the street and we got some odd glances on the way.

I felt as if I was inside a stranger's skin, looking through somebody else's eyes. Physically, I was in OK shape; the previous day had gone quietly. After the afternoon session in the Greenmount, I'd spent the evening in Mary's, with the wireless going, and reading the evening paper. Some guy down in Sailortown, below York Street, had murdered his wife and the headlines in the *Belfast Telegraph* were an inch deep. I had turned to the death notices: 'Reilly, Elizabeth. At home, after a long illness, wife of the late John Reilly. Deeply regretted by her loving sons John and William. Nearer My God To Thee.' As far as the world was concerned, I wasn't deeply regretting it. The notice had been placed by John, no doubt. Fair enough, in the circs.

I was in best blue order. The creases in my trousers were knife blades, the buttons were parade-ground Brasso'd, my shoes were black mirrors, my hat sat at exactly the correct angle. I walked smartly, carrying my right glove in my left hand and my head was up as I reached the first knot of mourners outside the house.

Among them was an air force corporal, a man whose face I knew. He came to attention and saluted. I was returning his salute as I reached the door and came face to face with John, peering out, looking for the clergyman.

The hall was packed with men, some in uniform, others in stiff serge suits. John turned and went into the parlour, pushing through the crowd. There was a cut on his brow, one side of his face was swollen and one eye was badly discoloured and stitched.

I went into the parlour behind him and stood by the door as the minister came in and took my hand.

'I have been told of the unfortunate events of Monday evening, Hugh. Put them behind you, go and take your brother's hand and carry this day through as friends.' He looked towards John hopefully.

'Just carry out the service, sir, will you, please?' John's voice was gruffer and more English than ever.

The rector looked sad. He caught my eye and I shrugged. His name was Pocock, he had a Dublin accent and a drip at the nose caused by too many funerals on cold days.

I stood against the wall, looked at the carpet, and the service began. I was standing at Mother's feet; the service lasted ten minutes and for all of them I was seeing her and listening to her voice.

On the last day of my leave she would say to me: 'Take another couple of days, won't you. Tell the man you weren't well.'

I remembered the day I brought Jackie Burgess in for lunch. He was a bomb-aimer who lived on the Crumlin Road. Was lost over Essen. Mother produced a special treat for us: 'I saved this for you,' she said. It was custard and prunes and we were sick looking at them in the air force. Burgess earned a DFC for the way he polished them off and then gave her a kiss.

Once, a girl called for me at the house. I'd met her at a dance and dated her. Mother sat beside me admiring everything I did as the three of us sat up for a cup of tea. 'Do you know what I like about him the most?' she said to the girl. 'It's his neck. He keeps it so nice and clean.'

As a boy, I picked the currants out of a loaf she'd baked. 'Who did it?' she shouted. Reply there was none, the three of us sat mute. 'If whoever did it owns up, I won't hit him,' she said. 'It was me!' I yelled, diving for the door, for she was too Irish not to hit me, promise or no promise.

In the coffin Mother's face seemed to have grown darker. Someone had fixed her hair where I had disturbed it and pulled it tightly back. It made her look almost Indian.

The clergyman had finished. She was dead and she was history. I found that I was feeling the little finger of my left hand. That's where I'd worn the ring that she'd given me, the one that the cabaret dancer had stolen.

The children of the district were sitting in a line along the kerb waiting for the coffin to be carried out. Many a time I'd done it myself. The two trestles were set out, the coffin was placed on top and the wreaths were brought out and laid on it. The children crowded round to read the cards.

I hadn't thought to send one. Damn.

People were taking my hand. The undertaker's man came over: 'You're the first lift, sir.' I followed him. He placed me at the head of the coffin, on the right. John came to the other side; Bill and Uncle Alec fell in behind. 'Just put your arms around each other's shoulders, and when you walk, walk out of step. It's easier, it doesn't rock,' he said.

I put an arm around John's shoulder and felt his on mine. Just before the coffin came between us I saw his bruised and cut face. Then, because I was taller than him, I took the heaviest share of the weight on my shoulder.

We moved off, John and I instinctively slow-marching, our feet shooting out at the correct angle, hovering fractionally before touching the ground. As we turned in to Duncairn Gardens I saw knots of onlookers, housewives wearing headscarves, some with wicker baskets, some holding children by the hand. Every window blind we passed was down. There, standing at the kerb, was Alma Conway, pulling her coat tight into herself against the morning chill, narrowing her eyes as she watched me. Behind Alma, against the wall, Mary Waugh watched too.

After about fifty yards the coffin was placed into the hearse. I was directed to a funeral car for the three-mile journey to Carnmoney. It had four pull-down seats at the back. I sat beside Bill; opposite Bill was a son of Uncle Alec's, which meant I was facing John. On the way we talked, the four of us, but John didn't once say anything to me directly, nor did I to him.

Carnmoney cemetery, under the black, intimidating slope of Ben Madigan, lay under a January morning mist. They lowered Mother on top of Dad, and after the burial service, the wreaths were laid on top of the grave. As the mourners bent over to read the cards, for form's sake, I did the same.

The previous night as we'd sat together I'd said to Mary suddenly: 'You know, after last night, people will think that I have no respect for my mother, but I love her and miss her so very much.' Minutes afterwards, Mary had risen and rushed out. 'Won't be long,' she'd said, 'I'll just get some wee thing for the supper.'

Among the wreaths was a beautiful spray of carnations

and chrysanthemums. The card read: 'Mother, I love you and miss you so very much. Hugh.'

In Owen Gallagher's pub on the Antrim Road John took charge. He went around the mourners in turn as we sat by the window that overlooked Belfast Lough and the green Holywood Hills beyond. A waiter noted the orders, but John's finger didn't point to me. When, finally, he turned to the waiter and said 'That's it', I rose, pulled a ten pound note from my pocket, went to the bar as the men watched in embarrassment, and gave the money to the barman. 'When this round's over, set one up from me,' I said.

I heard Bill and one of the men calling as I half ran out of Owen Gallagher's. Outside, a city-bound tram came along, rattling and swaying. I jumped it on the run, expertly, in the way I'd learned as a kid selling papers, and I rode it right to North Queen Street. I went into Mary's. She was in the scullery pouring tea. I thanked her for the wreath. Then she took me to bed. I think she expected me to cry, but I didn't. I just lay there, holding her for a long time. Then we went for it.

That evening Dicky Walters tracked me into Jimmy McGrane's.

'Your John was all delighted when you frigged off today,' he told me. 'Know what he said? He said: "No wonder he ran away. I'm surprised he had the skin on his face to turn up at the funeral at all." Know what one oul fella told John? Here's what he told him, he said to John: "Know this? Never mind anything else, if I'd a brother a flight lieutenant pilot I would feel proud of him", that's what he said, he said brothers fall out all the time but that guy must be good to be an officer, and he's the same as captain, and furthermore he looks like an officer. Know what I was going to do? I was going to thump John. They had to hold me.'

I gave him a long look. Jimmy McGrane had just brought the drinks to the table and he straightened and gave him a look as well.

'I *was*,' Dicky said, but there wasn't a big lot of beef behind it.

'You couldn't bate our Aggie and she's on crutches,' Jimmy said as he sat down beside us.

Dicky tried to tip him five bob for a three shilling round and got a severe lecture for throwing the money about that he'd earned so hard and sore.

'I suppose you're thinking of getting a bit of work,' Jimmy said to me.

'I'd better,' I told him, 'but it won't be easy; bombing military targets isn't a growing industry. But I'll tell you one thing, I'm not going back to the aircraft factory.'

'What would you like to do?'

I took a long drink and set the glass down. 'Know what I'd love to do? Write for the papers. Not as a reporter. Just write articles. But I've no chance. No education.'

'You've any amount of brains. And you can use words.' So could Jimmy; he could disguise it well, too. 'There's going to be big changes with Labour in government. Do you know, under that Beveridge Plan, every kid's going to have the chance to go to a grammar school, or even university.'

'Too late for me, Jimmy.'

'You've done one thing. Pilot will always be on your record.'

Jimmy went back behind the counter. Dicky began to hitch at his trousers and pull at the edge of his cuff. He cleared his throat: 'How's it going with your woman?'

'How do you mean, how's it going?'

'You'll be all right there.'

'Piss off.'

He took a swig. A thin wiggle of stout began to run down the side of his mouth. 'At least you know where you are, that way.'

'What do you mean?'

He screwed up his face, dropped his voice. 'I mean with the women. I suppose you've had them everywhere.'

I turned in my seat and my eyes burned two holes in him. 'Are you one of these squatters?'

When we were kids we used to go up the Grove, where the courting couples went. In the darkness, over the wide flat expanse of the playing fields, we used to crawl, like Red Indians, on the lookout for couplings. We saw plenty. The noise of the woman was the giveaway. But it was a dangerous game: if caught by the man, it meant a boot in the arse. Later, normal kids became normal men and gave it up. But there were also adult prowlers on the Grove, some of them men up to middle age. When we kids spotted one of these watching a heaving, panting pair of lovers, we would forego our own thrill and raise the alarm: 'Look out – squatters!'

'I'm not a squatter.' He was jiggling and twisting as if the fleas were at him. 'Look, don't be saying anything. Not to anybody, OK?'

I nodded, not really wanting to hear it.

'D'ye see girls? Well, I think I'm important.'

'You're important?'

'Can't do it. I've tried it a few times. No good. I'm important.' He was looking everywhere, in case one of the customers came close enough to overhear.

I laughed. 'It's common. You've been locked up for three years. You'll come good. Takes time.'

He shook his head. 'It's after what they did to me, just after I went LMF.' His voice was almost a whisper. 'They gave me jankers for a made-up charge. I'd done nothing wrong. They said I was insolent to a cookhouse corporal. Got seven days. Had to report in full kit to the guardroom every hour.'

I nodded: I'd had some of it.

'The first night, at ten o'clock, this big sergeant took me out to the exercise yard at the back. Like the rest of them, called me a windy bastard. Shoved a hanky in my mouth, took my trousers down.'

'Christ! That's a court-martial charge. Did you not report it?'

He smiled, gave a shrug. 'I went sick and the medical orderly said I was malingering, that I'd get the jail if I tried to bear false witness as he called it. That's when I put in for overseas. But there were six more weeks of it. It only stopped when I got my posting. But it has made me important, anyway. And you're the only one that knows. You're my mate.'

NINE

N EXT DAY AT LUNCH I said to Mary: 'I'll go out, have a few snifters, then we'll do the town.'

'No,' she came back, 'finish your lunch, and we'll go out this afternoon. You've clothes to buy. You don't want to run about in that outfit all the time, do you? Then you can step out this evening in your new clothes.'

She didn't call lunch dinner, as she'd done once, in the Belfast way, or the afternoon evening, or the evening night. I had to go away to learn that, but she'd learned it right here. We talked, she and I, just like the company we'd kept. What a difference six years had made. All around Europe, simple soldiers had picked up the same sort of words and brought them back home and the old local, lopsided, lovely way of talking was done for.

'Listen to this and tell me what you think of it, it's a little poem I wrote for you,' I said. Smiling into her eyes, I began:

> In my song of love the moon above has the music,
> The words are in my heart.
> My lips may be afraid to serenade you tonight,
> But the words are in my heart.
> The roses red in rhythm are swaying,
> And like my heart, they're tenderly saying
> My dear, I love you so, and even though I don't say it,
> The words are in my heart.

'I wrote that last night,' I said. 'Do you like it?'

She said nothing, just watched me closely, until the little smile appeared in my eyes. 'You bastard,' she said, lifting a cushion and whaling me with it, 'how many women have fallen for that?'

'Well, Joan Blondell did, when Dick Powell sang it to her. And you did, too, for a while.'

'No chance. What makes you think so?'

'Because you called me a bastard.'

After a bit, I said: 'All the same, I'd love to hear people sing a song that I'd written, or see people read and enjoy my words. It must be a marvellous feeling.'

She took me to a tailor's in Donegall Street, where I bought an oatmealy Harris tweed jacket off the peg, plus two pairs of grey flannel trousers. Between us, we also chose a grey-blue suit. When I tried it on she went narrow-eyed, womanlike, studying me. 'There's not a pick of extra on you and you should be big-made,' she said, 'so get a size that's going to be comfortable when the weight starts to go on.'

It was a fact that I was down to the bone. The life overseas had left me with kipper hips. We bought shirts and shoes, ties and underpants and then went into the Lombard for a drink, and as we sat with our parcels, she came with the Mona Lisa smile.

'What is it?' I asked.

'I've never done this before in all my life,' she said. 'Gone shopping with a man. Have you ever done it with a woman?'

I shook my head. 'And I never thought I would.'

'Christ on a crutch, Hugh, what a change there is in you. When I see you there, I keep thinking back to school, and those cocksucking teachers.'

'Oh yeah. You talked about that before. Imagine remembering me.'

'Remember you? I frigging fancied you. It was when I was thirteen, just before you left. I guess I must have been the only girl in the place who did. The others hated you. You were full of oul lip, and like a scarecrow, skinny, with a hole in the ass of your trousers, and a red nose. Your legs were the best part of you. You've still got lovely legs.'

'I thought it was only women who had lovely legs.'

'Don't you believe it. Ask any woman,' she said. 'One day you got such a beating for something or other. It was terrible. You were hammered right around the school, caned on the hands, the legs, across your back. In front of the whole school. And when it was over and you were nearly out on your feet, you still faced up to old Topcliffe. The look on your face! You hated the old bastard, and you wouldn't hide it.'

'Why did all that make you like me?'

'Because I hated the bastards too.'

'But they fed you, kept you bloody alive.'

'I know. That's why I hated them. When I was drinking that egg and milk in the mornings every eye in the class was on me. I had to take charity before the whole school. You know, all they had to do was let me take it in the teachers' room, by myself, but that never occurred to them. But you wouldn't take any shit from them. Every time you stood up to them I cheered inside, and every time they hit you for it I felt it.'

'Funny. I never knew that.'

'You wouldn't have been all that pleased if you had.'

'True, true. In those days I regarded all girls as informers.' I cocked an eye at her. 'Not like now.' I waited for her to fish for more, but she just gave me her level stare, nodded, and began to gather up her parcels. 'Come on, we've got a date,' she said.

'Who's this we're seeing?'

'Jack O'Hare. And don't ask questions. Come on.'

She took me to a bar in Corporation Street. Opposite the bar, the men were queuing to sign on at the buroo. When Mary asked the manager if she could use the pub phone to make a call, he seemed complimented; I was getting used to this by now.

I was surprised by the speed of O'Hare's appearance. He was five ten, broad-shouldered, sturdily built, wore a moustache and suited it, glasses with heavy black frames and a head of healthy black hair. He was a good-looking guy, but seen from any angle, he was a fixer.

'Hi, Hughie,' he greeted me. If my name had been Sam it would have been Hi Sammy, but his smile was warm enough. 'Any friend of Mary's.' He kissed her on the cheek.

'Jack's a clerk in the buroo,' Mary explained.

I was impressed. In our society buroo clerks were big stuff.

O'Hare sat down. 'So this is the candidate.'

'Candidate what for?' I looked from one to the other.

O'Hare said, after a glance at his watch: 'Mary says it'll be good for you to get a job.' He pulled a form from his pocket. 'I've already entered the names of two referees, both JPs. Fill the rest of it in and give it to me; I'm in Labour Control.'

Labour Control! Heavens above and the earth beneath, that's where they handed out the jobs. We once had a little guy at the bottom of our street who was in Labour Control and we just about jumped off the pavement to let him pass.

'I have no qualifications,' I told O'Hare. 'I left school at fourteen.'

He pointed to my pilot's wings. 'Don't be silly,' he said, 'Neanderthal man could do our work. They don't test civil servants to see if they're intelligent, it's to check that they're honest. Throw that form into me soon.'

'Where would I work?'

'Most likely in there.' He stood up, jerked a thumb in the direction of the buroo, waved to the two of us and left.

I looked at Mary helplessly. 'What's your next trick?'

'The word trick has a different meaning for me than for you,' she said.

'I know, I've been to the States. That's where I perfected the Dick Powell thing.'

That evening in the Royal Avenue Hotel lounge I noticed two women nearby who looked like prossies. It reminded me of something.

'I was talking to Dicky today. He says he's what he calls important with women. I was wondering if we couldn't rake up a good pro who could test his IQ.'

'IQ?' Mary stopped smiling at importance and looked puzzled.

'His importance quotient. I don't know if it's a common thing.'

'Look,' she said severely, 'if you were out with a lady dentist for the evening, would you spend time talking about teeth?'

I laughed. 'I think you're fabulous,' I told her, and I smiled to see such a good pro blush.

Dicky and Bill were sitting on the windowsill of Mary's house when we got back at midnight.

'This is going to surprise you,' Bill said, when we were in and settled, 'but have a guess who wants to see you.'

'Alma?' The minute I said it I glanced at Mary. She was setting teacups out; I thought that her eyes narrowed, on the word.

'Wrong.'

I sat in sham concentration: 'The Reverend Pocock, to heal the rift?' I was hoping to blitz the earlier mistake.

'I'd better tell you,' Bill said. 'It's Annie Longley.'

Now I was surprised. 'Me? Why me?'

Bill sneaked a look towards Dicky, who was spreading off-ration butter on white American bread.

'Never mind him, go ahead,' I said.

'Well, I'd guess it would be money.'

Mary's head popped out of the scullery. Her eyes were wide.

'Come here till you hear this.' I waved her in: I wanted Alma's name swept out of existence.

Bill said: 'She's a hopeless case with money. And our John knows nothing about it. She gives the kids in the street silver just for running a few yards for smokes for her. She has already borrowed four quid from me, but there's no sign of it coming back. One day Mrs Hagan round the back admired a set of saucepans she'd bought new and Annie just turned round and handed them to her. She loves to be loved. If you ask me, I think she's going to put it on you for a load of quid.'

'Cor blimey,' I said, 'and stone the crows.'

Next day I left the form into the buroo for Jack O'Hare, wandered around town, met a few guys from the past, and got back to Mary's at four o'clock. Dicky Walters was there, highly excited. 'That man that murdered his wife was up for hearing today in the Petty Sessions,' he said, 'and have a free guess who it is.'

I shook my head.

'It's the fellow that was on the beer with us that night in Mulgrew's. I knew there was something about that name. Dan Byrne. D'you not remember it?'

'No,' I said. 'But how do you know it's the same man? It's a common enough name.'

'Because' – he said it with a triumphant air – 'because I was there, at the Petty Sessions. Saw him, so I did. Same man definitely.' He was almost licking his lips. 'It's a weird sensation, looking at him, knowing his neck's for the rope.'

'You're a morbid wee bastard. I never would have thought it.'

He was smiling all over his face. 'I saw people being done in by the Japs. Sometimes they hanged them, sometimes it was chop chop with the sword. Oh aye. D'you see when they hanged them, well it was pure strangling. Now when Pierrepoint does it – '

'For Christ's sake!' Mary jumped up. 'I'm getting away out of this.' She stormed upstairs.

'This big Yank in the next bed to me one time told the guard that the emperor was controlled by the army. The Jap knew a bit of English and they'd often talked nice and friendly. But when the Yank said that, the guard blew his whistle and then led the Yank soldier out.'

I was listening, nailed to my chair, and Dicky's eyes were glowing as if he was on pep pills.

'The whole camp was paraded in the next five minutes, an officer made your man kneel, and then he cut the bloody head off him with one swipe. D'you know this? The blood shoots out for a yard.'

'Get back to the Petty Sessions,' I said, 'the Far East is frightening me.'

'He was only in the dock for about three minutes. Not a bad-looking cratur, just like you or me. D'you know what he called the RM? He called him your lordship, instead of your worship. Shows you – the poor bastard had never been in court before.'

'Are you going to be there to see the trial?'

'Wouldn't miss it. But I was telling you about Pierrepoint, the hangman. There was an ex-screw in Changi with us and he told me. From the time Pierrepoint goes into the cell till the trapdoor opens, it takes only twenty seconds. The condemned man's back's to the door, see? The screws offer the poor cunt a drink of whiskey. He reaches for it, Pierrepoint grabs him from behind, slaps the strap on his wrists, and starts pushing him to the execution chamber. Now, it's only a few feet away. It has actually been behind a cupboard, although the prisoner never knew it. Pierrepoint and his assistant push your man through the door and up the step . . . '

'Wait a minute' – I stopped the flow – 'tell me this: when did Dan Byrne murder his wife?'

'On the eighteenth of January, the night he was in Mulgrew's.'

'Christ. Was it before or after drinking with us?'

'After.' Dicky was loving every second. 'Just think, it could have been the drink we emptied into him that made him do it. He hadn't a bloody match, you know. He was sitting on his own in the snug when you landed in. Mary and me pushed you into the snug and from then on your man Dan was part of the round. We knocked him stocious. Then he went home and knifed the wife.'

'Knifed her?'

'Knifed her.' He was tasting the words as they came out.

I shuddered. Then, to get away from the implications, I remembered something. 'When I was at Aircrew Receiving Centre in London one of the cadets killed a local girl.' I nearly said prostitute, but it was a word now deleted from my vocabulary. 'The stupid bastard left his cap at the scene of the crime and the cops lifted him before morning from a billet near mine.'

'I mind that case.' Dicky's eyes were shining. 'He got topped. Pierrepoint was busy in the war, wasn't he? Just think,' he said, dreamily, 'your man Byrne's only got about three months to live.'

'That'll do.' I stood up. 'I'm going for a shower, to wash off that prison smell.'

Dicky went to the bottom of the stairs. 'Hey Mary,' he shouted.

'Yes, what do you want?'

'Can I stay here tonight? It's just for the one night.'

She came down into the kitchen. 'Why, what's wrong with your own place?'

'I got kicked out. You know the way I shout in my sleep? Well, this oul lad that lives there doesn't fancy it. He was in the last war and he says it's too noisy with the two of us shouting through the night.'

'No, I don't know the way you shout in your sleep and I don't want to. Anyway, you haven't had a bath since your mother gave you one. I don't fancy you in here. Go on out and go up and down the Duncairn Gardens and knock doors. Half of those houses were set out in flats to Free State workers in the war and a lot of them are away back to the South again. You'll get a place there easily.'

After he left, I showered and was towelling myself in the bedroom, thinking about Mary, when she came in. I threw off the towel and her eyes went mock big.

I used to know an air-gunner who told me that when he wanted to hold back and make lovemaking last out he would set himself a complicated mental algebraic problem. In this way, he managed to defer the earthquake until the moment when he found the solution. Trouble was, he was a brilliant mathematician.

Well, I had something that took longer than maths to help me take my time with Mary. It was called Dan Byrne.

TEN

M ARY AND I WERE sitting in the Royal Avenue again
that evening. So far, thank goodness, she hadn't
commented on my fondness for the juice, though God
knows she was no soak herself. I was pleased, too, that
she was giving so much time to me. It was a compliment,
since presumably it was costing her.

We were quiet and content. I was reading the *Belfast
Telegraph* when I heard Mary make a kind of tiny hissing
noise; I looked up. A man had just come into the bar, with a
woman.

The man was tall, hadn't any extra weight, aged about
forty-five, dressed in a brown suit. He had sallow features,

with the sort of dark hair that seems to manufacture its own Brilliantine, and he had long sideboards. They sat down in our view and in no time it was clear that he was having trouble in keeping his hands off her. In a matter of seconds, while chatting to her, he managed to touch her lower arm, her upper arm, and three inches south of her oxter. The woman looked uncomfortable, glancing around covertly. She wore a second-best coat, lisle-looking stockings, and a skirt best described as serviceable – she was obviously an ordinary housewife, and although her clothes were nicely filled she was dressed for fetching the messages.

Mary was giving him so much mackerel eye that I was surprised.

'Know them?' I asked.

'I know him, all right,' she said, 'and he's a leading shithouse.'

She told me his name was Leo Grogan. He was a money-lender, with two rooms in Donegall Street, nearby.

'One room is the office and the other room holds a bed-settee,' she said. 'The office is where he lends the money, and the other room is where he takes young wives who fall behind with their instalments.'

Leo Grogan was sitting tight-close to the woman, talking, using his hands.

'He brings them here to hand the loan over,' Mary said. 'Watch and you'll see.'

Sure enough, after the waiter had brought their drinks, Grogan said something to the woman, then from an inside pocket he took some notes. He rolled them into a tube, took the woman's hand, and tickled her palm with the money before closing her fingers around it.

I felt Mary shudder, and I nodded. 'It's all in the way he does it, isn't it?' I said. 'He's managed to put me off palm tickling for life. And the lady sure doesn't like it either.'

'He's a pig.' Mary's voice was filled with venom.

I was studying Grogan closely now. 'He can't go wrong, by his rules,' I said. 'After the grope session, she now knows the score if she skips payments. So he either gets his dough back dead on time, which is very nice for business, or if she gets into arrears, well, as he leads her into the other room, he can tell himself that she knew the score when she took the big lira. He's certainly making it clear enough.'

He certainly was. He was telling her a joke, and as he came to the payoff line he laughed and squeezed her thigh, just exactly dead smack clean on top of the button of her suspender belt.

Next morning Mary was out when there was a knock at the door. It was about half past ten. I was scribbling a few thoughts down in a writing pad. It was something I'd been doing ever since North Africa, writing little pieces and then throwing them away. I crumpled the sheet of paper into a tight ball and crammed it into the neatly laid fire and when I looked up Bill and Annie Longley were peering through the kitchen window.

Once inside, Bill was making faces behind her back as her eyes quartered the room, like a rent bailiff.

'I'm sure you think I'm awful, Hughie' – she was fluttering her eyelashes; she was very good at it – 'but I wanted to see you right away.'

'I'll shove off.' Bill was glad to escape.

When the door closed behind him Annie sat on the settee beside me. She looked around the room: 'I say, you're no mug. This is all right, eh?' Her smile was knowing, artful.

She sat looking at her knees, then she turned to me. 'What I say is this,' she said, 'you're a single man and it's a free country.'

I nodded: 'You're on the button there, all right.'

'My John's cut to the bone, but that's what I told him.'

'Well, it's certainly hard to argue against that.' I was intrigued. I wanted to see how she was going to turn this little gavotte into a business meeting.

'Is . . . you know . . . is she in?' She looked towards the staircase in a love-nesty kind of way.

'Mary's out.' I smiled politely.

'Did Bill give you any notion of why I was wanting to see you?' Her accent was poshed up, but not as much as John's.

I shook my head.

She tapped me lightly on the knee, and my radar did a search, but it came up with nothing except family. 'I'm in a temporary bit of a fix,' she said. She gave an off-centre smile. 'It's nothing, but John doesn't know about it, and you know what he's like.'

'Well, I don't know what he's like about money. That's what you're talking about, isn't it?'

'He's been sending me the money for, you know, the future, ever since we got engaged. There's a bit of a snag. I can fix it up. It's nothing, only I don't want him to know about it.' She wasn't one of those chancers who look away as the line's being shot. As she spoke, Annie Longley's eyes were on mine, holding them, locking on.

All of a sudden it dawned on me that this one had me taped. She'd known from the way I'd run out of the house and stayed away that here was a mother lode of guilt to tap into. It wouldn't have taken Freud to work it out, anyway, but I had to admire her neck.

80

'How much have you dropped?' I asked.

She swallowed, letting me see the swallow. 'I'm going down with him to buy some furniture, and to order my wedding suit. He has told me to draw it out of the post office book.'

'Does he never ask to see the book?'

'No, not up to now.'

'Doesn't he have any idea what should be in it?'

She shrugged: 'I suppose if he sat down and counted it he could get close, but he's very good, he's always left it to me.'

She was measuring me for the chop.

I stayed silent.

'Um, could you let me have forty pounds?'

I nodded, watching her eyes for the quick stab of annoyance. It came on the instant: she could have made it sixty, maybe more. I rose and was searching my jacket for my cheque book when the door opened and Mary walked in, her cheeks pink from the January morning. Annie got up, straightening her skirt and the advantage in every single way was with Mary. She looked great. She was a soufflé, to Annie's egg with no salt. Claret versus cooking sherry.

'This is Annie Longley,' I said, 'she's our John's intended.'

Mary stood cool while Annie carried out sweep patterns up and down, in and out and through her. Mary smiled, said how do you do, put her basket down and they shook hands.

Mary slid out of her coat, and made the tiny kitchen a stage, in her soft white angora sweater, neat, deep blue skirt, fine denier nylons and platform-soled, ankle-strapped white shoes. 'I'm sure you haven't had a cup of coffee yet,' she said. 'I'll go and make us all one.'

Shaking her head, Annie said no thanks, it was all right. Grabbing her coat, she waited awkwardly as I went to the table, wrote the cheque, held it until the ink dried, and handed it to her.

Mary opened the door, I put my arm around her shoulder, and that's the way Annie saw us as she left with the forty quid.

Back inside, I said: 'I'm sorry about that. When you took me in, you took the whole bloody crew on board.' She didn't look as though she minded, but I owed her an explanation. 'Drama piles upon drama. Annie is up to the diddies in debt, and John knows nothing about it.'

'When are they getting married?'

'Not long to go now. One of her problems is buying her wedding suit.'

Mary made a face, but said nothing. She went into the scullery and began to empty the basket.

'Hey, those are the sort of shopping bags you see in the Hollywood pictures,' I said.

Mary drew out a large tin of Virginia ham and a packet of ground coffee. From the other bag she took a white loaf. What she had there was grub straight from a Yank PX store.

I studied her. In these iron ration days she looked as appetising as the Virginia ham she'd brought. I wondered if she'd been . . . well . . . out in the line of business. There was no reason why not. It wasn't necessarily a night job. I lay against the scullery entrance, watching, as she started the coffee percolating. Every now and then she would look up and meet my eyes, and my eyes were easy with hers. She was relaxed, and when I was with her, so was I.

As we were sitting together drinking the coffee the knocker banged. It was the postman. Mary came back with a letter in her hand. 'On His Majesty's Service,' she said, 'and it's addressed to you, care of me.'

'Well, I won't argue with that form of address,' I said, opening it. 'I am to present myself at the Tech at ten o'clock in the morning for a written competition for a temporary post in the Northern Ireland Civil Service.' I checked the date. 'In the morning? They don't allow much time for swotting up, do they?'

'You'll be all right,' Mary said.

'I'll have to take it easy tonight,' I told her, 'this is like a boxer before a big fight. The better he performs with the nookie the worse he performs in the ring.'

There must have been a couple of hundred candidates sitting the test. There were uniformed officers and NCOs from all branches of the services, including majors – one in a kilt – and squadron leaders. All after a job that paid four and a half quid a week, and ten shillings off that for tax and stamp. It wasn't a great time to be out of work.

I wasn't hopeful. Clearly I had to beat lots of these guys to get a job. But at least the arithmetic was money for jam, and the English was straightforward. Since it was a competition, I took care with the English, but it was no problem, I enjoyed doing it, covering six foolscap pages on the essay in the hour.

I showed Mary the questions, afterwards. She sat, hugging her knees as I went over my answers and told her what I'd written in the essay.

'Sounds great,' she said, in a faraway voice, reaching over and picking at my shirt button.

'At school I could have licked anybody at English,' I said, 'but that was our school, Mister Topcliffe's Establishment for the Sons and Daughters of Swanky Ragmen. Some of those guys today had the classy look about them.'

The last button eased out.

'Mm . . . but did Jack O'Hare say that they would get the job?'

'No, I suppose not.'

The shirt was being pulled out of the waistband.

'Well then don't talk rubbish and get on with it. Do what the boxers do when the fight's over.'

ELEVEN

I WAS CALLED FOR an interview only three days after the written test. They must have been in a hell of a hurry for clerical assistants. There were three men behind the table. They looked tired. Full ashtrays and empty teacups on the table told of long hours of talking. The one in the middle opened up with my war record, another one asked me what I knew about civil service work.

'Nothing,' I told him.

'How do you know you'll be able to manage it?' he asked.

I was flummoxed, until I remembered something. 'I was a staff officer in charge of personnel at Air HQ Bari for nearly a year,' I said. 'Do you think that might help?'

They looked relieved. 'How would you feel about working in Belfast Employment Exchange?' the chairman enquired.

I told him it would be fine with me, and they all smiled and bade me good afternoon and told me not to book any holidays or anything, for I could be sent for soon.

'What about going to Dublin to celebrate?' Dicky Walters suggested.

Mary wasn't on for it, but I thought it was a great idea. I'd never been to Dublin in my life. In fact, I'd never even been over the border.

'I think this is going to be one of those men things,' Mary said. 'I don't feel like trailing after you two around the pubs in a strange city. Anyway, I don't like those bastards down there.'

I'd never thought of the Free-Staters as bastards. My Uncle Sammy loved to go to Donegal and Sligo and when I was a kid his descriptions of these places made me want to see them, but I never had. I'd known lots of Free-Staters in the air force and noticed that, when they met, North and South nearly always came together as big mates. But Mary lived in Orange Duncairn Ward, the place chosen by Lord Carson for his title. She'd had no Uncle Sammy and hadn't knocked around with any southerners.

'Their government sat back and did God curse all in the war and let us take the pasting along with Britain,' she said, and I couldn't argue with that. 'Anyway,' she finished, 'they all worship statues.' So that finished that debate.

There was a bar on the train and we stood up to it, lowering bottles of stout, talking to a merchant seaman from Dublin. His ship was in Belfast and he was going down for an overnight with the wife and kids. By the time we reached Dundalk we were feeling warm and chummy.

The train stopped. 'Take a look at that,' said Dicky, grabbing my sleeve.

On the platform a long snake of people stood, mostly women. At the head of the queue two uniformed men were stopping some and allowing others to board a train that lay beyond their table.

'It's the customs,' the Dubliner explained. 'They're taking away the stuff that the northerners have bought in Dundalk.'

As we watched we saw an officer empty the contents of one woman's basket on to the table. He tore open a flat package; it was cooked ham, maybe a pound weight. The woman, kitchen house all over, in a headscarf, argued with the man, pleaded, then walked slowly to the train shaking her head.

Dicky had the window down. He stuck his head out. 'Man but yer a great pack of shitepots,' he yelled, 'give the woman her bloody ham, ya miserable gets yis.'

The customs officers looked up; so did the queue of northerners on the platform. At first they all smiled at Dicky. Then some woman in the queue shouted: 'That's right, son. They're a lot of bloody bastards.' Next, the whole queue started shouting and crowding around the table. The woman who'd lost the ham turned, came back, and in the mêlée lifted it off the table and made for the Belfast train. The roar from the platform was doubled by another. Windows had opened on our train and the Dublin-bound passengers had joined in.

I felt out of things and shoving Dicky out of the way, I shouted: 'Anyway, you all worship statues.' It was just like an air force mess party.

'Hey, frig off, Hughie,' the seaman said, mildly. 'I worship statues too, you know.'

'Burn them out,' Dicky screamed.

'Overthrow the government,' I screamed.

'Give the woman her ham back,' the seaman shouted.

The customs men had been pointing to us and shouting directions to someone. There were heavy footsteps in the corridor, and suddenly two Free State peelers, about six and a half feet each, burst in. The three of us were pushed, punched, dug and generally manhandled on to the platform, a whistle was blown and the Dublin train steamed off without us.

We were taken across the footbridge, past the cheering queue; Dicky gave a boxer's salute to the crowd as, tripping and stumbling, we ended up in the customs office.

'We're British subjects, and we demand to see the ambassador,' Dicky shouted.

One of the policemen belted him clean across the face with the flat of a hand that looked like a shovel. We sat, the three of us, in the office, while the police took statements from the customs men. After about an hour, we were taken out to the station forecourt and driven to the barrack in a blue police van, with the strange Garda sign on its side. In the barrack the three of us were flung into a cell that smelt of vomit.

We weren't worried, Dicky and I, but Thomas, the merchant seaman, was. There was a good chance that he might miss his ship. I shouted for the guard.

'That man comes from Dublin. He's innocent, and if he's not back on board his ship in the morning it'll sail without him,' I said. 'Why don't you just prosecute us and let him go. After all, he's one of your own, why should he cause trouble? It was only Dicky and me who did the shouting.'

The guard went away. We sat for a good couple of hours and by that time the drink had died in us, good and proper. Eventually we were brought out and led to an office upstairs. On the way I muttered: 'Leave the talking to me.'

Behind the desk was a man of middle age with rank badges on his shoulders.

'This is a jail offence, do you know that?' He spoke in a disinterested voice. 'What you're looking at here is six months.'

We looked at six months, then at him, then at each other.

'May we speak, sir?' I asked, in as timorous a voice as I could manage. These people were the spit image of the RUC. The wallop across the gub suffered by Dicky proved it, so attitude was everything. What was needed here were signs of blue funk, plus a proper appreciation of the majesty of the police. 'We were the worse for drink, sir,' I said weakly.

'You were that,' he said.

'And we're very sorry, sir.'

No reply.

'And, sir?'

He inclined one eyebrow fractionally.

'Sir, this chap here had the bad luck to be in the bar when we were lifted. He's from Dublin and he works on a boat and it's sailing in the morning. Sir.'

'Is that right?' He turned his eye on the seaman.

'Show him your discharge book, Thomas,' I said.

Thomas handed it over.

The policeman lifted his phone and spoke into it.

'You can go,' he said to Thomas. 'That leaves you two. Seemingly only one of you can talk. Talk to me now about him.' He pointed at Dicky.

'D'you see that man there, sir,' I said, 'well he's not long out of a Jap prisoner of war camp. Three years, sir.'

'Is that right?' he asked Dicky, who nodded. 'Where was the camp?'

'Changi,' Dicky replied.

'How did you come to be captured?'

'We walked down the gangway of the troopship practically straight into prison. Singapore had just about collapsed when we tied up, sir.'

'Hm.' He studied me: 'And what's your story?'

I stood meekly. 'I have none, sir.'

'Were you not in a Japanese jail?'

'No, sir, thank God.' I considered crossing myself, then scrubbed it.

'And you're not a seaman about to miss your boat?'

I shook my head. I liked his tone; my spirits were rising.

'Well tell me about yourself. You were in the forces, by the look of you.'

I was surprised. 'I was, sir.'

'And what did you do?'

Dicky took the initiative for the first time. 'He's a flight lieutenant pilot, so he is, sir.'

'Oh' – his head went sideways – 'and what did you pilot, then?'

'Wellingtons, Mark Ten.'

He sat forward: 'Ever heard of Thirty-seven Squadron?'

'Yeah, they had Wimpeys too, in Italy.' I'd forgotten the servility. 'At Foggia.'

He picked up the phone and spoke again. When he put it down he said: 'You're being taken to the station. You'll take the six fifteen from Dublin back to Belfast. I want you to get into that buckin' train and get the hell out of buckin' Dundalk, right?'

At the door I turned: 'Who did you know in Thirty-seven Squadron?'

His head was down over some papers: 'Never mind. Bugger off.'

TWELVE

'JEEZ, TAKING THE GARDA on in the Free State!' Jack O'Hare's eyes were shining. He had called to see me at Mary's next evening, and we'd all repaired to the Greenmount. 'And nearly starting a riot at the station. Brilliant.'

Our cuteness had been filtered out of the version that Dicky had given him and I hadn't done anything to put it right.

'It's more than anybody I know has done.' O'Hare was delighted. 'Wish I'd seen it.'

Dicky said: 'Well, I'll tell you one thing, they know all about the Prods in Dundalk now, all right.'

'I think you're like a lot of school kids,' Mary put in. 'You'll notice that the only one to do the sensible thing in the whole tale was the woman who got home with the pound of ham.'

'I'll tell you why I called.' O'Hare was cleaning his glasses as he spoke. 'You'll be getting word to start in Corporation Street very soon.'

I didn't want to spoil his party by telling him that I already knew. 'Thanks for your help.' I pointed my pint towards him.

'You got it on your own merits,' he said, 'all I'm doing is getting you posted to Corporation Street. I think you're the right sort for it.'

A couple of days later Bill called at Mary's to see me. 'I've got terrible news for you,' he said. The look in his eye hinted that he didn't feel as bad as he sounded.

'Yeah?' I said. 'Leave nothing out.'

'Right. John has applied to join the civil service.' He leaned back on Mary's sofa the better to enjoy my reaction. It was expressed in one word.

'I thought you'd be pleased.'

'How far has it gone?'

'He's up at the clergyman getting his name for the form, then he's going to some RUC man who was in the regiment.'

Poor bastard. No JPs, like me.

That night, as Mary gawked, I got down on my knees beside the bed: 'God, you know I'm an atheist but you've got me out of scrapes with night-fighters in the past, so I'm asking you for this special one: please, please let our John get the job in the civil service because if you don't, it'll be the story of the commission all over again, and John's liable to go batchy for ever and ever, amen.'

Corporation Street was the biggest labour exchange in the United Kingdom, maybe even in Europe. Only unemployed men signed on there. The signing counter was all of fifty feet long. It was also chest-high, to make it hard for the workless to get their hands on the box clerks. I wasn't long in finding out why.

I was put to work with a Free-State-born, ex-RAF clerk called Walworth. Every fifteen minutes about a hundred and fifty claimants were admitted to the building, and, of these, about twenty signed on at Walworth's box. He himself stood holding a flat board in his hand, which was used to mark the place of each claimant's file when it was brought out for signing. The files were in long, narrow boxes kept beside the counter. Walworth was responsible for Box 54 – unskilled labourers.

Halfway through my first morning a man in his fifties arrived. He threw his UB40 in front of the clerk. It spun and came to rest the wrong way round. Walworth pushed it with the edge of his board.

'Turn that card round, mister.' Walworth didn't even look at the man as he spoke, he just waited, staring down at the card.

The man's face flushed. He was tall, neatly dressed, with well-kept hands. 'What did you say?' he asked.

Walworth's voice was low and level: 'I can't read that card; turn it round.'

'You turn it round, it's your bloody card.' The man's hands were gripping the counter, his fingers were white. Behind him, the queue watched silently.

'D'ye see that wall over there?' Walworth was pointing to the white-tiled wall by the door; the claimant turned his head. 'Go over there and put your arse against that wall, mister, and you wait till I call you.' The box clerk picked up the card and handed it back.

The man sucked in his breath, his face changed, he began to lift one hand.

'If you as much as swing that arm you'll get prison.' Walworth still wasn't excited; his voice, harsh with the accent of one of the border counties, was steady and controlled.

'You bloody arrogant, fascist bastard . . . ' The claimant stood, trembling with rage.

Behind him, another man plucked at his sleeve: 'Go ahead and wait over there, mate. He's right, you'll get the jail if you touch him. It's automatic jail.'

The man turned and slowly made his way to the wall.

He stood there for three hours, until half past twelve, then he was beckoned forward. With exaggerated movements he placed the card the right way up in front of Walworth, who expertly slipped the file out, stamped it, and turned it around for signature. The man signed, tight-lipped, and went out.

'And that,' said Walworth to me, 'is how you handle big heads.'

'Just like the wogs in Egypt,' I said.

'Dead on.'

After a week I took over Box 54. I smiled at the man who'd been stood against the wall. 'If you like you can birl your card so that it ends up the wrong way round,' I said. He smiled back, I stamped his file and he signed the docket.

When he left I winked at the next one in line. He'd been watching with interest. He laid his UB40 down and tapped me for a quid. I told him to get stuffed.

'There you are you see,' he said, 'you new ones always start off decent, but it doesn't take long for you to get like all the rest.'

THIRTEEN

D ICKY WALTERS GOT A surprise when he came to sign
for his dole: I was his box clerk. I wagged a finger at
him: 'This won't do, war heroes trailing down to the buroo
twice a week, it's undignified. I'm afraid you'll still have to
call in on Thursdays for your twenty-six bob, but at least I
can spare you from coming here on Tuesdays.'

And so he signed his docket in the Greenmount on
Monday evenings and I slipped it into his file on Tuesday
mornings. But Dicky wasn't all that happy about it.

'You're taking the whole dignity out of the job,' he said.
'The previous box clerk once grabbed my hand and inspected my fingernails. He saw paint there, because I'd been

helping Herbie Irons to paint his motorbike. "I hope you're not working for a painter and lifting the buroo," your man said, "from now on I'll be watching your nails." Now that's more like the way a box clerk should behave.'

Jack O'Hare took tea with me in the canteen each morning. 'I was telling them in Glengall Street about that carry-on of yours in Dundalk. The PM was tickled pink,' he told me one day.

'Do you mean to say that the top Unionists were talking about me? The Prime Minister? Sir Basil Brooke?' My eyes were sitting out like dog's balls.

He was smiling. 'I'm on the Unionist Council, for dear sake, Hughie. I'm an Orange Order delegate.'

'Do you help to run the country?' I knew nothing about the Unionist Council.

'Well, I help to select candidates, and I attend the party conferences and, in between, discuss party policy,' he said.

While I was thinking that it was no wonder he carried so much thump – he was only a clerk but every one of the bosses seemed scared of him – O'Hare handed me a brown envelope.

'Tell me what you think about that, Hughie.' he said as he left.

I opened it and began to read, but the reading didn't last long. It was an official form. Across the top, in bold type, were the words Royal Ulster Constabulary. It was an application to join the B Specials. I folded the form and put it in my pocket.

I was over in the pub opposite the buroo at lunch time when O'Hare joined me. I got him a drink, and as he started on his sandwiches he said: 'Well, what do you think?'

I took the envelope from my pocket and gave it back to him, shaking my head.

'No go?'

'No go, thanks all the same. Are you a B man yourself?'

'I'm a head constable.'

I raised my eyebrows, impressed.

'Tell me this, Hughie, and I know you'll take this the right way, is it for any kind of political reason you don't want to join?'

'Jack, listen,' I said, 'I have no politics, none. But I have to tell you two things: one, I detest patrols and guard duty and sentry go and everything of that sort. On airfield guard in the war we only had to do two on and four off, and it nearly drove me batchy. Those two hours took two years to go in. Peelers and B men do all night out on the beat. My arse on that for a way to put the time in.'

'And what's the second thing?'

'It's this: when I was a kid the RUC weren't any friends of ours. They moved us on when we stood in a group, they lifted us and had us fined for playing football in the street. At the street corner they shoved and needled men who had fought in the trenches until one of them shoved back, and then they beat him up and threw him into the Black Maria. I don't know whether they've changed their way of going or not, but I know this – the ordinary people haven't changed their opinion of the peelers, and I don't want anybody to feel that way about me.'

O'Hare pushed his glasses up with a forefinger: 'You know, this concerns Ulster's future.'

'In what way?'

'This way: I'm talking about the Free State and the IRA.'

'Oh, that.'

'It's all right for you to say "Oh that", but this is the real war, Hughie. Some day it's going to come down to it between us and them. The Taigs want us to hell out of it. When the British left the South, a hell of a lot of ordinary Protestants were burned out and chased over the border. There is no Protestant working class down there now. None. And there never will be. That's what the Taigs want to see all over the island. Then they can make a whole palaver over the tiny wee group of middle-class Prods that are left, and pass it off as tolerance.' He dug a pipe out of his pocket, put it in his mouth, began to thumb tobacco from his pouch. 'OK, the B men are doing ordinary police work now, but you know and I know why we're really here, it's to protect what we have when the balloon goes up.'

I nodded. 'You're probably right, you know more about it than I do. Certainly I met plenty of Free-Staters in the Raff but none of them was a Prod; there seems to be an acute shortage of our sort down there. But even so, I'll have to pass on this one.'

He drew on the pipe; he was one of the few young men who looked natural smoking one. 'Never mind,' he said. 'It's my job to recruit the right sort, when I can. You would have been dead on. We need brains as well as the other thing.'

'Maybe I might have failed the blood test, anyway, if you know what I mean.'

O'Hare smiled. It was a politician's smile that faded as he began to speak. 'I know all about your blood. You're a Prod, with Prod parents. That makes your blood all right. This is not Nazi Germany, you know, where the blood was checked right back to the grandparents. I was happy to help you to get a job here when Mary Waugh asked me. You'd have got the job anyway, on your exam and interview, but I was there if I'd been needed.'

'By the way, Jack,' I said, remembering, 'I've a brother who has put in for a job. His name's John. Could you do anything for him?'

He shook his head, leaning over to tap the pipe out on to an ashtray. 'Sorry, Hughie. I've got stronger calls on me.'

As I made my way back to work I was thinking that John was going to fail the exam that I'd passed. As the paratroopers used to say just before they jumped: here goes nothing.

At Mary's that night Dicky Walters launched straight into the report as soon as he sat down on the sofa.

'Dan Byrne and his wife Briege were told to get out of their room in Sailortown if they didn't pay up their rent.'

Mary and I looked at one another resignedly.

'He'd drunk his day's pay,' he continued. 'When he got home Briege kicked up holy hell. She came at him, he hit her a dunt, she went for him with a knife and he got it and polished her off with it.'

'Where did you get all this gen?' I asked.

'I was down in Mulgrew's. It's common knowledge along York Street.'

Mary said: 'Is Hugh's name going to come into it, for giving him the drink?'

'No, don't be daft. But what do you think? Do you think he'll escape the rope?'

'It could be manslaughter,' I said.

'How?'

'Well, if he killed his wife trying to stop her from killing him.'

Dicky waved the possibility away: 'Do you know what'll

finish him? The fact that he was full drunk. Judges are sudden death on working-class men getting full drunk.' He smiled: 'Don't worry, Dan Byrne'll take the morning stroll.'

Mary jumped up. 'You weird sonofabitch. What's that to us? Go and jerk yourself, you stupid bastard!' She went to the door and opened it.

As if he was a balloon man with a puncture, Dicky's whole body sagged. 'I was only telling you.' He looked at me. 'It's only my wee hobby, isn't that right, Hugh?'

'That's right,' I said to Mary. 'Hanging, and Pierrepoint; it's only his wee hobby.'

But it didn't save him. Mary pointed to the door and Dicky walked out, bowing his head to Mary, as if she were a Jap prison guard.

FOURTEEN

O NCE WHEN I WAS sitting in my tent in North Africa, almost numb from daytime tedium, I sat and watched a scarab beetle climb all the way from the sandy floor to the top of the tent pole. I stood, picked it off the cord, carried it outside, and set it down on the sand. I laid it upside down, with its head pointing away from the tent, to disorientate it. As I watched, it struggled upright, turned, made its way to the entrance of the tent, found the pole, and climbed it again to the top.

I removed it, took it further away, past three tents, laid it down, covered it with an inch of sand and observed it. Up it came to the surface, and after a look around, it headed back, dead on track, past the three tents, to mine. Then up it went to the top of the pole, where I left it in peace to whatever the hell it was up to. I wondered whether entomologists knew that scarabs carried built-in homing devices. If not, then maybe I could apply to have that part of the insect's system named after me.

It helped to punch in the long, non-flying hours. I took to watching scorpions: they weren't as dangerous as they were made out to be. Their sting was nasty, but not fatal, although it was said that an air-gunner down in the Nile Delta had died from multiple scorpion stings. He was blind drunk, the story went; when they found the scorpion it was down inside his shirt.

But the scorpion had an insect foe that didn't give a good God's curse for reputations: this was the scorpion beetle. Often in the night hours I sat alone and watched one of these beat the tar out of a scorpion, expertly avoiding the sting like a judo champ.

I caught flies and fed them to a lizard – always the same lizard, I had bombed its tail with a blob of Stephen's ink. It wouldn't eat dead flies, only those lightly stunned with the swat and still twitching. This led me to wonder whether the world knew about this side of the lizard's feeding habits. I'd get my name in a natural science book yet.

But the star of the show, when I was playing the game of monotony, was the praying mantis. Of all my actors of the insect world, this was the one to remember. To see a mantis catch a fly was a privilege. The speed of the snatch was incredible, then it would eat the fly like a toffee apple on a stick.

And then there was their sex life. Talk about living dangerously. If the male mantis wasn't off the mark and airborne double quick after mating, he ran the risk of getting the toffee apple treatment, as well. I saw many a one gobbled up because he stuck around too long, dreaming, after having his jollies. As we liked to say in the RAF, he shouldn't have joined if he couldn't take a joke.

I sat down and wrote a nice tight eight hundred words about the insects, and I sent it to the editor of the evening paper, with a note saying: 'This is submitted for publication, if you like it.' That was on a Monday. The following Saturday evening Jimmy McGrane straightened up from reading the paper, glanced at me over the top of his glasses, and bent closer over the page. Then he carried the paper to where I was sitting listening to a couple of pigeon fanciers talking about the Penzance race.

'That must be you,' Jimmy said, spreading the paper out in front of me. It was open at 'Saturday Miscellany', a weekly collection of writings. Across the top, over the lead piece, was the heading: 'Actors of the Insect World, by Hugh Reilly.'

They hadn't changed a word. That pleased me. Later, Mary saw it. I was amazed at what she did, to show how pleased she was.

On Monday, still pleased, I was at the counter, signing claimants. It was ten thirty in the morning. A tall thin guy appeared before me.

'A brother of mine signs with you at four thirty,' he said, 'and he wants to come at the same signing time as me.'

I looked at his card, searched for the brother's unit in the late box, and switched the unit over. 'There you are,' I said, 'no sooner said than done.'

'Just a minute.' The voice came from behind me. It was one of the supervisors, a purple-faced, bossy bastard, name of Foster. He had obviously overheard the exchange.

'Why does this brother of yours want to sign earlier?' Foster asked.

The claimant looked confused.

'Well, tell him that once these signing times are worked out they can't be changed, all right?' Foster reached past me and took the papers.

'No, just a wee minute there,' I said, 'hold the horse by the head.'

Foster's face grew even more purple, the claimant looked down at the ground, and the queue behind him pushed forward eagerly, sensing drama.

'The thing about it is,' I said, 'I'm the one who does the signing. If it suits me to change one man's time, where's the harm?'

Foster took my arm and led me to his desk nearby. 'If you're not careful I'll run you in to see the manager,' he said. 'You'll do as I say, right?'

'Are you not going to give this man a reason?' I asked, 'or me either, come to that?'

'Go and do what I tell you.'

'Bullshit.' I turned back to the counter. The claimant went away, half smiling, half worried.

Two minutes later a clerk new to me slid into my place and prepared to take over. 'You've to go to the manager's office right away,' he said. His glance was darting sideways to me, as if he was taking in every detail before I was put away.

The manager was surprisingly young to be running such a huge dole office; he looked to be about thirty-five.

'Mister Foster here, your supervisor, has laid a serious complaint against you, Mister Reilly,' he said. He was studying me with considerable interest, and without evident rancour.

'If that's serious, he's had a remarkably trouble-free life,' I said, and the beginning of a twinkle came to the manager's eye.

'He ordered you to do something and you refused?'

'He ordered me to do something, I asked him for his reason, and he was the one who refused. Instead of giving me a reason he threatened to run me in – his words – to see you if I didn't do it. In the event, I didn't run, I walked in.'

The manager played with a paper clip. 'In fact, as I have already made clear to Mister Foster, the decision as to signing times is, indeed, your own, since this affects no one but yourself.'

Then Foster spoke. 'If we let these people sign whenever they like the place will be unmanageable. That man's brother only wanted to sign early so that he can go and gamble the money on the horses.'

I laughed in disbelief. 'Well, so what? Isn't it his own money? Sure what business is it of ours what a single man does with twenty-six shillings? God knows, it's not as if he's going to start a run on the pound, or anything.'

The manager was openly smiling now. 'I get the feeling that you can take this job or leave it, Mister Reilly,' he said, 'but that's your business. In the meantime, let me tell you that, as an ex-officer, you should know that there's a limit to the extent to which you can suck up to the other ranks, so watch it.'

He was thorough; he must have been reading my file. He waved a dismissal to a partially mollified Foster, and signalled me to stay. 'Tell me,' he said, 'was that your piece in the *Telegraph* last Saturday?'

I said it was.

'It was very nice, very deftly written. You should write more. I enjoyed it very much.'

I left feeling simultaneously bollocked and praised, but the praise had won by a length.

FIFTEEN

I WAS DATING CLAIM units, thumping away with my rubber stamp, when the phone on my desk rang. I picked it up, a voice spoke, and I was transformed into a high-tension battery: it was Alma Conway, my cousin.

'Could I speak to Mister Reilly, please?' She was hesitant, low-voiced, unused to the phone.

'Speaking,' I said cheerfully.

'Is . . . is that you, Hugh? It's . . . ' her voice almost faded away, ' . . . it's me, Alma.'

'Sure I know it's you, Alma. It's smashing to hear your voice.'

'Hughie . . . I was just wondering how you were.'

She was just wondering how I was.

'Where are you?' I asked.

'I'm in a phone box in Corporation Street.'

'What are you doing there? Is anything wrong?'

'No. I was down the town and I just . . . just thought I would like to talk to you.'

'Listen, Alma, I'll go out and see you. Where exactly are you?' She told me. I jumped up and tore out of the buroo. Kiss kiss, Alma.

In the little snug of Mulgrew's pub I closed the door behind us and held her and kissed her. It was a very good, frank, candid kiss, a kiss that talked its head off. Then we sat down. I didn't ask her why she'd come looking for me; I just smiled and waited.

'I had to see you,' she said.

'Well, I'm glad you so decided,' I said, but she was so miserable that I jacked in the smart approach. 'You're looking great.' I was ogling. She had opened her coat to reveal a cream light woollen jumper that was needing every ounce of tensile strength it could summon up to hold her bosom back.

'I think it's awful, you living with that woman.' Awful was one of her favourite words. Too much awful would get on my wick, but certainly not yet.

I could see our family in her face. I could see some of myself in it. Her eyes were the same brown, her hair the same black; her cheekbones were high, like mine. I was vibrating. It was the family thing: if it was incestuous, well, four cheers for it.

'Look, meet me tonight at seven. Castle Junction, at the kiosk, all right?' I said.

'All right.'

I went back to the buroo, dreaming about tight blouses on Catholics. I saw no faces as I signed the workless. They passed in front of me, insubstantial figures, indistinct images. Then, suddenly, no longer indistinct. Bloody crystal clear, in fact. It was my brother John. Oh that I had wings like a dove.

He'd wanted so much to be commissioned in the war that now he was dressing like an ex-officer. He wore a tweed suit, fawn and grey, and his shirt was country check. On his head he wore the sort of cap that cavalry officers wore at Sandown Park races, and although I couldn't see his feet I just knew that he was wearing stout brown ankle boots. He was the country gent, come back from the war, to take over the management of the estate from the wife.

He was second in the queue and his eyes were everywhere but on me.

'Oh, hello,' I said, when his card dropped in front of me. There was no reply. I riffled through the claims, found his, and shook my head at the realisation that I had received, processed and filed it without noticing that it was my own brother's. Just as well, anyway: waiting for the encounter would have made the day so far seem like a month.

John was embarrassed, and showed it more than I did. He had to stand and wait, whereas I had all these little movements and procedures to give the impression of coolness.

When I gave him the docket he took my indelible pencil, signed his name in his round, innocent hand, and pushed it back to me.

'That's it until the same time Thursday,' I said breezily, and he turned and walked away, with his shoulders straight and his arms swinging, and I saw that he was, indeed, wearing brown, good quality, ankle boots. I could almost have cried for him. Then I remembered Alma and snapped out of it.

After work I called into the Greenmount for a drink before going to Mary's. Dicky Walters was sitting, half cut, by the window.

'I'm running the poker school tonight,' he told me.

He'd been living in a flat on Duncairn Gardens for over a week; a bare room in a house full of characters who, according to Dicky, were on the run either from wife maintenance orders, the income tax man, or the military police for wartime desertion.

'I didn't think that those screwballs in your place were sociable enough to play poker,' I said.

'I'm not talking about that bunch' – Dicky's eyes were lit up – 'I'm entertaining some real sharks. They can't get a place for their regular school, so I've volunteered.' I was puzzled and he explained: 'I provide the cards, and I shuffle and deal. I make tea, fetch drink and cigarettes, and do general dogsbody. I was down in the Capstan Bar today and I heard your man Leo Grogan and that hard man of his saying that they didn't like the house where the poker school's based at present – a wee kitchen house somewhere, too small, and kids about the place – and I told them that I had this big room and nobody there but myself, so I'm elected.'

'Leo Grogan?' I sat, snapping my fingers, then I got him: 'The moneylender?'

'That's him. He's a regular poker player, gambler generally, goes across the water to see the big fights, that kind of thing.'

'He was put up to me as a bit of a no-user: watch him, Dicky.'

'Other way about, Hughie. Leo Grogan'll have to watch me.' He laughed, renewing the Guinness-trickle down the sides of his mouth.

On my way to Mary's I was shaking my head. He was a headcase and no mistake.

'What's on tonight?' Mary asked. I had just come downstairs after showering and she sat watching me as I tucked the tail of my shirt in.

'I've to go to a union meeting. What are you doing yourself?'

'I'll maybe run over and see Marita.' She had a roster of friends with names like Marita, Carmella, Estelle; she didn't talk about them, and I didn't ask. 'I can't see you as a union man.' She was taking in every centimetre of me.

I was uneasy. 'It's just curiosity,' I told her. 'There's a poker school in Dicky Walters's place and I might look in there later.' Then I kissed her and left.

Alma was waiting. I took her arm, thankful for the dark evenings of January. Downtown Belfast was looking good, well lit up. People were standing in Castle Place, craning up, reading the words that the electric news was pushing on lighted bulbs around the screen above Leahy Kelly's, the tobacconist's. There was a damp chill in the air and many of the women wore thick ankle socks. On all sides, night life was bustling. There was a queue for a Robert Taylor picture in the Royal Avenue cinema, and the cafés were filling up.

At the four corners of Castle Junction stood the last survivors of the hundreds of wartime street women who'd serviced the GIs. They were gazing brightly around; the Yanks had nearly all gone, but there were still plenty of ex-servicemen with cash gratuities to blow.

112

I had to work hard to keep the thrill of the evening's promise a length ahead of the guilt that I felt about two-timing Mary, but once we were safely on top of a trolley bus, and were swishing through the traffic, and the knee-talk started with Alma, things became easier.

We got off on the Lisburn Road and I walked Alma to the Margrave Hotel, a licensed place, one of a row of handsome four-storey Victorian houses set well back from the road. Inside, I rang the bell at reception. I knew what I was doing. A school friend, Bertie Neill, worked here as the live-in porter. I'd met him a few days earlier. 'Any time you want a bit of peace and quiet with a woman it'll be no bother, Hughie,' he'd said.

Bertie appeared, and palmed the quid I slipped him. He showed us into the bar, a cosy little four-table room with nobody else there. He served our drinks. 'I'll just fix things up for you,' he said.

As we waited I said to Alma: 'This is brilliant, isn't it?'

She gave a nervous smile.

'You don't regret it, do you?' I asked.

She shook her head. 'No, but, oh, I don't know how I feel. I just want to be with you, that's all.'

'But what?'

She was having trouble in finding the words. I helped her out: 'The way you saw it, we would meet a few times, talk a few times, go for little walks, maybe, and hold hands. Then, somehow, without any of us bringing the subject up, we'd make love, and walk out together, defying the world to part us. Was that the scenario?'

She was defensive. 'Well, if it was, what's the matter with it?'

I took her hands and said: 'Alma, do you want to get into bed with me tonight or not?'

She glanced at me anxiously, saw that it wasn't an ultimatum. I was smiling. The beginnings of a smile came into her eyes, too.

'Look,' I said, 'face it squarely: you fancy me like the clappers. You're on fire. Your loins ache for me. Why can't women come right out and say these things? Tell me that you want tonight, upstairs, to end up in a fireworks display. Alma, you're busting for it, old thing.' By then she was plain straight laughing. We were lovely and lascivious. So now we could leave it and pick up the romance.

I said: 'Do you remember the times when you brought messages to our house and I used to see you safely out of Protestant territory?' She nodded. 'Well, when I turned fourteen, baby, the things I did to you in my fantasies.'

By the time Bertie came back my voltage was strong enough to light up Castle Junction. He handed me the key to the room.

There was a double bed, high off the floor, with a heavy, embroidered coverlet. A marble-topped table, with jug and bowl, stood by the wall; there was a dressing table with three mirrors, and two wickerwork, well-cushioned chairs. The room was pleasantly warmed by a gas fire; the thick carpet was going to be soft on bare toes.

I helped Alma to undress and was glad to see that the experience wasn't unhinging her. That afternoon I'd been worried; she'd shown the classic symptoms of the virgin, but the conversation downstairs had reassured me. Now, seeing me hypnotised by her bare breasts, she smiled, followed my eyes, and, like some women, looked down critically at herself, wondering what men saw in them; glad of it, whatever it was.

We stood naked, baked together, in a spot of my choosing, so that I could see us in two of the mirrors. My hands were holding her fingers, to counter an urge on her part to flay the skin off my back with her nails. Then I led her to the bed.

I began to think of her old man, Uncle Sammy, and what he would think if he could see us now. It helped to spin things out. Christ, she was strong. But I was stronger. And the two of us started in and it was a murdering match.

Next I thought of her mother, a warm, kind-hearted woman, but what would she say if she knew? That line of thinking was good for four shifts of position and emphasis.

Lastly, I fell back on an old and trusted routine: I went slowly and carefully through the cockpit check before take-off. Then we rolled and we were airborne.

When it finally ended, what we had there was Hiroshima. It took us half an hour to get over it. And then, of course, what with the nice comfortable bed and everything, and this thing that I had for cousins and Catholics, we started in again. This time it was no Hiroshima, but Iwo Jima wouldn't have been out of order as a comparison.

After seeing Alma on to the bus I walked to Dicky's place. It was midnight; the poker players hardly looked up as I pushed the door open and entered. The room was full of cigarette smoke and the smell of stout and stale chips. The screwed-up chip papers lay in the middle of the floor. Dicky was sitting, low down, on a cushionless, dilapidated sofa backed against one wall, and the table was pushed tight against the sofa. On ordinary chairs around the table the three other players sat. They were a good foot higher than Dicky.

I went to the cupboard by the cooker in the corner and found the tea makings. There were only three cups and two milk bottles, all dirty. I washed up, made the tea, and carried three cups over to the visitors, with bottles each for Dicky and myself. Then I stood leaning against the wall watching the game.

Leo Grogan was studying his cards. His poke amounted to around thirty quid in notes and coins. The other two were worth less than a tenner apiece, but Dicky was nicely loaded. After giving me a suspicious glance Grogan put his hand face down on the table. 'Your three quid and up three,' he growled. The other two packed. Only Grogan and Dicky were left.

Dicky shifted the Woodbine to the other side of his mouth. For the moment he was Edward G. Robinson. He held Grogan's glare impudently. 'You've got a bet there, fella. Your three and up five.'

Grogan stared at him with distaste. 'I thought you were supposed to just deal and make the tea,' he said. 'I'm still trying to work out how you came to be in the school.'

'I'm in the school because the other ones said it was OK,' Dicky replied, squinting through his cigarette smoke. 'Are you in or are you out?'

After another long look Leo Grogan tossed his hand in. Then he stood up. 'Come on, Bucksie,' he said. A burly, rubbery-faced guy stood up, pushed his chair back. He was about fourteen stone, a long scar from his scalp ended in a drooped eyelid. The two of them stared down, half mockingly, at Dicky. Grogan looked around at the room, lit only by a single bulb hanging from the centre of the ceiling. 'This'll do all right for the school.' He pointed a finger at Dicky: 'You've made yourself a couple of bob, but you'll need more than you started with tonight to play in my company. Next time you're the tea boy, and for that you get a shilling a game and whatever the winner likes to bung you.'

Dicky was happily gathering up his money and shuffling the cards. 'That's all right, son,' he said, 'we'll see what the school says about me playing, but I'll see you when I see you. Mind the stairs when you're going out.'

Bucksie leaned towards Dicky: 'You're a bit of a mouth, aren't ye?'

This was where I came in; Dicky had turned to me. 'He's not, but I am,' I said, 'I'm a mouth. Is it a mouth you're looking for?' I had stopped lounging, and spread my feet a little. I let the bottle slip through my fingers until I was holding it by the neck, and all the time I was staring into Bucksie's pig eyes.

'I'll be seeing you,' Bucksie said. He was watching my hand on the bottle.

'Happy to oblige,' I answered. To prove it, I treated him to a happy smile as he and Leo Grogan turned and left.

The other two players let out their breath. One grabbed his coat and fled, but the other one, a man of about fifty, with a bookie's clerk look to him, eyed me in admiration. 'Christ but I enjoyed that,' he said. 'It was worth the twelve quid I lost.' He nodded to me and left.

Dicky pushed the table back. 'C'mere,' he said, 'till I show you something. Take a look under there.'

I had to get down on my hunkers to see, but when I saw what was there I stood up so suddenly that I bumped my head on the edge of the table. 'Merciful God!'

To the underside of the table Dicky had fastened a stretch of strong elastic, and tucked into the elastic, held clean out of sight, were several playing cards. I took one out. It was from a pack that was identical to those lying on the table. 'You're insane.' I stared at Dicky almost stupefied. 'Were you drawing from those cards during the game?'

117

He drummed with the flats of his hands on the table: 'I didn't put them there for decoration, mate.'

I looked again at the table layout. Now I could see why Dicky had taken the cushions off the sofa. With the others raised so far above him, they couldn't see him fiddling underneath for the extra cards.

'I learned that one in Changi,' he said with a wink.

'Promise me you won't try it when the proper school starts.' I was in earnest. 'They'll bloody kill you.'

'Don't worry, Hughie, I know a whole lot more wheezes than that. I can look after myself.'

I walked down Duncairn Gardens worrying about Dicky, feeling guilty about Mary, and thinking that the storm clouds were bound to break if Alma and I went public.

SIXTEEN

I SIGHED AND MARY stirred and stretched and turned to me. I knew one thing for sure: I knew all the street tricks, but I was no good at double-crossing women. Although I had time on the clock for affection, I kissed Mary, eased away from her, and got up.

'What time is it?' she said. Her voice was usually enough to get me going in the mornings; it was low, husky, sexy, her eyes were half-closed and her arm lay across the place where I should have been. She raised her head to see the clock. How the hell any man could walk away from her baffled the brain, but I was doing it. I showered, dressed, and went to work, leaving Mary behind in quiet mood. She was no noodle: she'd have noted the magneto readings.

I was well past thoughtful myself when I sat down to morning break in the canteen.

'Congratulations,' Jack O'Hare said.

'What for?'

'You've got a writing style.'

That lifted me somewhat. 'You saw that piece in the paper?'

He slapped me on the back. 'I don't know if you know it or not, but it's some achievement to get into the "Miscellany". It's usually the bookish ones who are published there. In fact, you're the first working-class writer I've known who's managed it. And no wonder: it was entertaining and easy to read.'

I could have taken any amount of this but he went on to something else: 'Hughie, could you do a job for me? A writing job? I'll pay you for it.'

'What is it?'

'It's the Unionist monthly magazine. I'd love to have an article in it but I can't write well enough. I've got the ideas, but when I try to set them down they come out like lumpy porridge. I'd be too scared of what the educated ones in the party would think if I ever saw print.'

'And what way do I come into it?'

'Look, I've got some notes at home and you could knock it into good strong reading. If you want to know any extra stuff, you can talk to me.'

'I'll have a crack at it.' Writing was writing. It would be good practice.

'What's the fee?' he asked.

I thought for a bit and said: 'How about two quid?'

'How about ten, Hughie?'

I whistled. 'Means that much to you, does it?'

He nodded. 'I'll tell you some day what it means to me.'

He was so keen on moving the thing along that he got the bus to his home in Finaghy, three miles away, and brought the papers back with him. It was a quiet afternoon for me and I sat studying the blots, corrections, scratches and scribbles.

He wanted to warn Unionists against putting the British government's back up unnecessarily. Across the water, socialism was strongly supported: Westminster would expect the Unionists to administer Northern Ireland taking this into account. Soon there would be radically new social benefits for the old, the poor and the sick, a free health service, state allowances based on the size of the family, sick pay was to be taken away from private insurance companies and taken over by the state – in Northern Ireland terms, in short, in O'Hare's view, the Catholics were going to be the main beneficiaries and he was anxious that Stormont should not be seen as begrudgers.

It was a piece that would have to be carefully written and from the outset I was caught up in it. The finished product would have to give the appearance of welcoming the welfare provisions due to take effect fully in 1948, but in appearing to welcome its application to the whole community, to Protestants and Catholics, it would also have to serve as a warning to the backwoodsmen in the Northern Ireland cabinet against using the normal precautions against fraudulently drawing the dole, or claiming sickness benefit, while working, as a means of bearing down on Catholics. Down that road lay the risk of Westminster looking again at the convention that Stormont's internal affairs would not be raised in London. I put the notes in my pocket, wishing I could do this sort of work all the time, instead of taking a march-past of the workless twice a week.

That evening I took Mary to the Classic picture house. 'It's *Fantasia*, a cartoon thing,' I told her. 'Do you like classical music?'

'Hm, some of it. I don't know much about it. It's all right to go and hear a full orchestra, but I must say I can't take it for long on the wireless or on the gramophone. I'd never buy a record of it.'

It would have been with one of the colonels she'd have listened to the full orchestra, I thought. In the time I'd been with her, I don't think she'd seen any colonels. She had a telephone upstairs and it had rung sometimes, but her low conversations hadn't resulted in any dates that I knew of. For myself, I'd only been to one concert, one opera, and one ballet, all in Rome. I'd loved the atmosphere, but, like Mary, with a few tuneful exceptions, like *Swan Lake*, I could otherwise take most of it or leave it.

I settled in beside her, as Leslie Chadwick finished his selections on the Classic Wurlitzer organ. The cinema darkened for the main feature. We were very still.

I put my arm around Mary for Ponchielli's 'Dance of the Hours'. Then came *Night on the Bare Mountain*, and as Disney's bizarre animation appeared on the screen and the first notes filled the cinema, I closed my eyes, tightened my arm around her. She turned to me and I kissed her, and behind us a woman said: 'Imagine, at their age.'

'What's wrong?' Mary whispered, but I kept kissing her until Mussorgsky's music ended and the opening notes of Schubert's 'Ave Maria' began, then I stood up, held my seat back to let her past, and we went out into Castle Arcade.

Walking through the narrow entry to the Castle Tavern, Mary said: 'That was funny sort of kissing in there.'

'What sort of funny?'

'Like . . . like kissing me sorry.'

I stopped and turned to her. 'Mary, I was with somebody last night.'

A tiny question mark of red hair had fallen on to her brow, and she fed it back into place, staring into my eyes. 'Who was it?'

'Alma Conway, my cousin.'

Mary's eyes closed; she shook her head.

'It's serious.'

She was winding the wisp of hair around her finger.

'Will I take you home?'

She suddenly sighed and began to button her coat high to the neck. 'I managed before you came along,' she said, 'and I'll manage after you. But life sure is one fuck-up. Let's go and hang one on.'

And so we did. We didn't say another word about Alma, but Mary grew more American in her speech as the session wore on. It was only in noticing this that I realised how she'd lost so much of it over the time we'd been together.

I woke up on Mary's settee just after six. Beside me, on the cosy rug, was my suitcase, packed. Without washing, shaving, or even looking around for a last time, I closed the door of Mary Waugh's house quietly behind me and walked through the grey morning to Dicky's flat.

SEVENTEEN

'D O YOU FANCY GOING down to the Nightshift Club?'
I said to Dicky. I'd hammered him up out of bed
and we were sitting in his cheerless living room. In as few
words as possible, I had brought him up to date and he
was delighted about it all, because it had brought him a
flatmate. 'The club opened at six. It'll be going full belt
now.'

We walked to York Street and hopped a trolley bus to the
Junction. Five minutes' walk over Queen's Bridge to a point
opposite Station Street and we were there. The man on the
door liked Dicky. All club doormen did. They'd been tipped
handsomely out of his POW back pay.

It was an experience to leave the quiet, early morning street and enter a packed and noisy pub. Dicky was hailed by a group near a roaring coal fire. They made room for us. I ordered whiskey and stout, Dicky asked for a pint, and the drinks were brought to us by a cheerful waiter with a flattened nose.

'Let me introduce myself,' said a little fat guy of about thirty-five, 'I am Doctor John Hughes. If you ever need a doctor's opinion, I'm your man.'

I only just managed to hold my eyebrows down. He looked like a hobo, in a greasy jacket, shirt worn to a frazzle, and trousers shiny with spilt drink.

Dicky nudged me: 'He's not bullshitting; used to be a doctor, your man.'

Hughes pointed to his companion. 'This is Henry Jackson, man of the law.'

Henry Jackson looked more like an orphan of the storm. In his early forties, he was long and thin and had a long thin nose. He wore an overcoat that had no buttons. Under the overcoat was a shirt, but no jacket. He had spent so much time sitting in pubs with the palms of his hands on his knees that both legs of his trousers were worn right through, revealing bony knees in sore need of a wash.

'Used to be a solicitor, your man. They're two mates,' Dicky said, at which both men nodded proudly. They glanced, with delicacy, towards their almost-empty glasses and when I signalled to the waiter they beamed at Dicky, delighted at his choice of company.

'What about your work?' Dicky asked me. I gave him a short and pungent reply to that one, and began drinking for effect.

The Doctor and the Lawyer had neatly created a

firebreak, isolating the four of us from any others in the vicinity who might be short of the price of a drink. On first sight of the new shiny fivers I produced to buy the liquor, two tongues licked two sets of lips and two pairs of eyes shone with new life. Gradually, as Dicky and I kept the waiter busy, the rest of the noisy scene faded into the background, and only the four of us existed. Before the day had properly begun, I wanted the blinds drawn on it.

These two characters suited my mood. I listened as the Lawyer told how he had embezzled the proceeds of the sales of three houses and had done time in Crumlin Road jail for it. 'They had to fetch me from Bristol,' he said proudly. 'Got two years at hard labour. If I hadn't conducted my own defence I'd only have got one year.' We nearly peed ourselves laughing.

Then it was time for the Doctor's story. The cause of his downfall was greyhound racing.

'What's wrong with that?' I was amazed. 'What's the matter with a bit of a flutter?'

'That's what I told the General Medical Council, and do you know what they said? That it's one thing to have a bit of a flutter, but it's something totally different to supply the dog trainers with both sorts of drugs – the slower-downers and the hurrier-uppers. To which I replied that I didn't need drugs to slow the beaten favourites: all I had to do was back them.'

'How do you get by, the two of you?' I wanted to know.

'I sell things door to door,' the Doctor said. He bent and from between his feet he produced a flimsy cardboard case, the sort that small children got from Santa at Christmas time.

'What's in it?' I asked.

'Nothing,' the Doctor said, 'I haven't the money to buy the french letters.'

126

'Frenchies door to door?' I couldn't believe it.

'If a woman answers, or a man over twenty-five years old, I ask if they need any knives sharpened, but you'd be amazed at how many young lads'll buy frenchies. The half of them can't get to use one, but just having the packet to show their mates makes them feel good.'

'What's your line?' I enquired of the Lawyer.

He shook his head. 'Nothing. I just tap.'

'Who do you tap?'

'Everybody. But mostly the punters around McAlinden's pitch in Castle Arcade. There's a good class of punter there, quite a few greyhound bookies as well, doing bets at the horses. Most of them remember me when I was going well.'

'Had a big house and a car,' Dicky put in.

The Lawyer inclined his head, acknowledging it as a compliment.

As usual, Dicky brought the talk around to murder. 'I love murders,' he said, with his gape-mouth smile. 'I love watching the one in the dock, studying him. That's a brilliant case going on now, that Dan Byrne. Do you think he'll get the works?'

'If I was laying odds on it' – the Doctor's eyes were half shut as he made the calculation – 'I'd make him six to four on to hit fresh air.'

We looked to the Lawyer for an expert opinion. He placed the tips of his fingers together: 'Speaking as someone who specialised in property conveyancing, mind you, not criminal law, and having read only the press reports, and bearing in mind that we only have the preliminary hearings to go on, if I were put to it, my professional opinion would be that your man Dan Byrne will be buried in lime before the end of the jumping season.'

127

After that the talk got on to other things, from the nationalisation of the coal mines, through the riots out in India, to the Nuremberg war crime trials.

'I'm telling you, there'll be some hanging going on out there soon,' Dicky gloated. 'Pierrepoint's arms'll be sore, shoving them Germans on to the trap. Imagine that big fat git Goering. If it was me, I would only give him an inch of a drop and throttle the bastard.'

'Dangle while you strangle,' the Doctor said.

'You know what Goering'll be shouting, don't you?' I volunteered.

'No, what?'

'The suspense is killing me!'

'You can't be serious, you must be choking,' the Lawyer roared.

The club closed at ten o'clock, as the pubs opened. Laughing and kidding like teenagers, the four of us made our way towards the nearest bar. There we found the darkest corner, so that we could hold on to the night time.

Next morning I awoke early, drank three cups of tea, and reflected. I'd taken one day off work without ringing in. I was still in no mood for work so I went out and bought the papers and sat on an electricity junction box reading the news until it was past nine o'clock. Then I rang the buroo and asked for Jack O'Hare. 'I was on the tear yesterday,' I told him, 'and I don't feel like going in today either. Can you let them know?'

'That's all right, Hughie, you can take two days' casual sick without a doctor's line. You're actually supposed to ring in before noon on the first day, but seeing you're new it'll be OK.'

'Thanks. I'll maybe do something on your magazine piece.'

'I'll tell you what, I'll call over this evening and see how you've got on. Where are you staying?'

I told him and hung up. He was certainly in a hurry for results.

Dicky's flat was like one of the many billets that I'd lived in in Italy. I slept on a mattress on the floor of the bedroom, Dicky and I shared a bathroom and toilet with the other occupants, the legion of the lost, and we spent our time in the dreary living room, with its rudimentary furnishings, and the bare, lino-covered floor in dire need of a scrub down with disinfectant.

When I got back Dicky was up and about. We opened a tin of beans, toasted some bread on the grill of the ancient roaring gas cooker in the corner, and afterwards I pulled a chair up to the table, told Dicky to keep quiet, and started work.

It was finished in two hours. Doing paperwork with a pounding hangover wasn't new to me, I'd done it for all the months I was with Air HQ. It looked all right. I seemed to have reproduced in readable language what O'Hare was carrying around in his mind. I was so pleased to have finished it that I went to the phone and told O'Hare that it was ready for collection. I took it to the Greenmount and he arrived all expectation.

'I can't think of a title for it,' I told him. Indeed, I'd tried half a dozen before giving up.

'Don't worry about that,' he said, 'that's the sub's job, not yours.'

Sub: I took a note of the term. He left his pint and his sandwiches neglected on the table as he read my longhand closely. I was pretending to read the paper but, to my own surprise, my eyes were rarely off him as he frowned over the five closely written sheets. I watched as he finally folded the pages and sighed with relief when he put them into an inside pocket and smiled. 'Brilliant,' he said. 'Bloody superb.'

I was pleased at his reaction for my own reasons, but the grin that spread across his broad face was so bright that I had to mention it. 'Will this do you a lot of good in the party?' I asked as he unpacked his lunch.

'Look, Hughie, I might as well tell you. There's one thing you have to get if people are to know that you're of any kind of consequence. This'll help me to get it.'

'And what's that?'

He pulled the pages out of his pocket and slapped them on the back of one hand: 'JP after your name, that's what.'

I was puzzled. 'Justice of the Peace? Does that not mean you have to sit in the court and that kind of thing? Anyway, I didn't know that you got JP through working for a political party.'

He was excited. His finger shot up to the bridge of his glasses. 'It's mostly decoration. You get to meet royalty when they visit, and people come to you for references, that sort of thing. Only once in a blue moon you might have to preside over a hearing – if the police want to lay formal charges in the middle of the night, or the like of that. But there are JPs who never see the court. And yes, a big lot of them got it through politics, local government councillors and so on. For God's sake, Hughie, there's a man who got JP for running messages for the secretary of the party. He washed the secretary's car outside HQ, and he even papered and painted the secretary's house once.'

The vehemence in O'Hare's voice was proof that he lived in unionism: no other world existed for him. He fished two fivers out of his wallet. 'Thanks, Hughie. Money well spent.'

I had plenty of money but those two fivers meant more to me than the rest, down to the last ha'penny. It was a fee for written work. I could earn money from writing. It was a marvellous feeling.

But a whole mixed grill of feelings awaited me when I got back to the flat. Dicky handed me a letter: 'Annie Longley left that just after you went out. She went to Mary Waugh's looking for you and Mary sent her round here, with that letter. Annie Longley said she'll be back.'

I looked at the letter, turned it over; the address was typewritten, on the flap at the back was a red seal, and in tiny white letters on the seal were the words 'Today's News Today.' I opened it and took out a folded statement. A cheque fell out. It was for three guineas. On the billhead from the evening paper were the words: 'Hugh Reilly, Esq.' and then 'Article: Insects. £3.3.0.'

I kissed the cheque. This was real earned income. And there'd be more. I wanted to rush to the table and get it going.

I pictured Mary's little welcoming house, and I remembered how she'd taken me in when there was no need to. That night on York Street she could have let me run past, to wherever I was going. And there was everything that had followed, all given by Mary.

Then I thought about Annie Longley coming back. What the hell did she want?

Dicky was sitting on the sofa, surrounded by papers, letters, postcards, snapshots; an opened suitcase lay on the floor. He was holding something which I recognised at once, a faded linen-backed book, blue, well-thumbed, with the words 'Observer's and Air-Gunner's Flying Log Book' in bold print on the cover. He handed it to me: 'Would you like to see it?'

131

I turned quickly to the operational entries. They covered some of the roughest raids in quite the roughest part of the war – strikes against airfields and installations in Norway, the tactical reaction to the German breakthrough in France in 1940, leading up to Dunkirk, then, after that, raids on the invasion barges, shipping in the Channel ports, and raids on German warships in heavily defended ports like Bremen and Hamburg, all in Bristol Blenheims, and all in daylight. On some of those raids nearly all the Blenheims were lost. And where an aircraft got back damaged, it was very often the gunner who'd been damaged most.

Dicky had done a hundred and twenty operational flying hours, half of them in murderous flak or under pursuit from fighters. The last entry read: 'Ceased flying. LMF. Sgd L.W. Coote, W Cdr.'

I looked at some of his photos – the usual aircrew collection, crews in flying gear grouped together before take-off. Nobody was ever in the mood for posing after landing. I handed the log book back. 'Nobody can take that away from you,' I said. Then I went to the table and started to write some more.

I'd thought of another wheeze to further my journalistic training and I tackled Jack O'Hare about it.

'Why don't you move into the trade-union caper?' I asked him.

He looked at me blankly.

'Listen,' I said, and I outlined my idea.

In the war people like Jack O'Hare and I had worked for buttons. As a sergeant pilot, I had earned about four and a half quid a week, less tax; O'Hare's pay as a petty officer writer in the navy had been three guineas a week. Not very much. On top of that, money was deducted from our pay under the Postwar Credits Scheme. The government was doing the same to civilian workers. We were all supposed to get our money back when the war ended, but we didn't fancy our chances.

Now, with the war won, here we were, people like O'Hare and me, working in the civil service for four and a half quid a week, less ten bob tax.

'If I were a trade unionist I'd help lead a movement for better pay than that,' I told O'Hare, 'it's exploitation. In the services we didn't expect decent money, but there's a Labour government in now and we servicemen helped put them there. I've written a good long piece for the union magazine, arguing for a fair day's wage for a difficult day's work. These national health regulations are not easy. They take a bit of learning. Why should we do it for soldiers' pay?'

He looked doubtful until I played my strongest card.

'If you were a trade-union figure, wouldn't it give you added swipe on the Unionist Council? You'd be the only bloody one who could claim knowledge of shop-floor thinking.'

I sat waiting. He considered it; then he saw something in it; then he liked it; finally he loved it. I pulled some pages from my pocket and laid them on the table.

'It's all there,' I told him. 'Fire it in to the editor of the union mag. You've seen it. It's murderous, all full of in-talk about efficiency bars, pay-straddlers, analogues and increments. That piece will put some life into the bloody magazine for a change. It's strong and there's no flash union-talk in it, because I don't know any. The editor will jump at it. Use it to get into the union branch here, work at it, go to the conference as a delegate, get on to the executive council, you'll eat them for breakfast, with your background.'

O'Hare's eyes were rolling like the tumblers in a slot machine. He lifted the pages. 'I'll have a go at it.' He was almost ready to kiss the piece I'd written: 'You know who runs the frigging unions here, don't you?'

I shook my head.

'It's the Taigs,' he said. 'From top to bottom, it's the Taigs.'

'There's more where that came from,' I murmured, 'the usual rate will do.'

EIGHTEEN

T HERE WAS A BOOKSHOP on Donegall Place called Mullan's, a pleasant place, shining with books, and where the assistants would talk about books without once giving the impression that they were there to sell them. I was a popular customer there, and not surprisingly, since I was God's gift to the shop – a guy who hadn't long discovered Maugham and who had only just heard of Robert Graves, so, simply to make me an average reader, Mullan's had a pension stretching before them.

I nipped smartly round there from the buroo during a slack spell. I went intending to buy *The Painted Veil* and came out with *The Mysterious Universe* by Sir James Jeans, hoping to bolster my atheism, having opened it to read that life is nothing but the carbon atom. I stepped out on to the busy pavement and ran into Mary Waugh.

She was loaded with parcels. I nearly knocked one out of her hands.

'Oh, hello,' she said, when I'd pulled myself together. It's a good sign when a woman says 'Oh, hello', not using a man's name, and it's not a great sign when she just says 'Hello', so I was glad of the Oh.

It put me in a talking mood. 'Did you ever know that you and I would be nothing if it weren't for the carbon atom? It's all in this book, and you are one of the greatest collections of carbon atoms the world has ever seen.'

She liked it, so I cashed in. 'Come and have a coffee with me,' I said, and when she hesitated I added: 'I've nipped out of work and it'll only be for ten minutes.'

Together we walked down to Bridge Street to the ITL café. I wondered what the people passing might think of us as a couple. A swirling, downtown breeze was blowing my hair all over the place and I kept running my fingers through it to make it lie down. My shoes needed cleaning, my tie was, as usual, loosened and pulled to the side, and there were no creases in the trousers that the breeze was pressing close to my long legs. Beside me, Mary, with shoulders that didn't need the fashionable, high military look, wore a maroon coat that folded over and belted tightly to show waist, hip and bosom lines emphatic enough to revive a man taking the last rites. Under it I could see the top of a deep blue dress, with dipping white lapel things, and on her neat and tidy feet, ankle-strapped leather shoes, purple, to tone with the coat.

'That's a nice outfit,' I said.

She laughed. 'Thank you, a compliment from a Belfastman is something special.'

136

'How do you think I'm looking,' I enquired.

She looked over and up. 'Mmm, about the usual.'

'By which is meant?'

'You need attention.'

We sat over coffee.

'I've written another piece for the paper,' I told her, 'and I'm leaving the buroo, so one of these days I'll be doing nothing all day but write. Write and drink. Maybe I'll move on from these article things and write a real story.'

'I'm certain sure you'll write stories some day. But why are you leaving?'

I remembered that it was Mary who had first thought of my going there. I shouldn't have told her I was leaving.

'It's depressing, Mary, and it's too much like the air force, you know, rank and promotion, and arse-licking in all directions.'

'Well, I hope you'll be all right, Hugh.'

'Thanks for all that you've done, Mary,' I said suddenly, but when the words were out they sounded like a dismissal.

She looked down at her coffee. I didn't push it.

'Look,' I said, 'do you want a job?'

She was surprised: 'What?'

I was anxious to get away from the thank-you business. I mentioned Jack O'Hare and the Orange and purple strings being pulled in Labour Control. 'He's going to be a justice of the peace, and a senator, and I'm his ghostwriter. He thinks I'm great. Would you like a job? I'm going to get our John one. And also Alma Conway . . . ' I stopped. I was watching her. ' . . . I'm not going to see her any more.'

'Oh.' That was all. She was looking at me directly enough. It wasn't as if she was hiding pleasure, or anything.

'I'm not going with anybody, I don't want to, but I'd like to stay friends with you.'

She began to gather up her parcels. 'You are friends with me, Hugh.'

I left her to the door; she was going right, I was going left. I didn't know whether to take her hand or kiss her on the cheek. In the end I just said: 'Bye bye, Mary Waugh', and I winked at her as she smiled. I watched her walk away. I stood on the pavement and watched until she reached the end of Bridge Street. Turn to me Mary, turn and wave to me.

She reached the corner, then she stopped, looked back up Bridge Street, and smiled. I smiled back. My hand was holding my hair down and with the other one I waved, and it was lovely, the way that we parted friends.

Foster, the supervisor, wasn't too chummy when I resumed my stand behind the desk. He tapped me on the shoulder and spoke in a low voice as I signed the claimants. 'You're supposed to get somebody to inform the office within the first hour when you're going to be absent.' Satisfaction showed in his eyes. He could see that I was the sort to keep giving him good cause for complaint.

I was signing busily as he spoke. I stamped a docket, slid it over to the next claimant, and asked: 'Didn't Jack O'Hare fix it for me?'

'He did, but only after a day had passed. I had a lot of trouble getting somebody to sign your box. You'll still be hearing from establishment division, and never mind what Mister O'Hare said.'

I walloped the date stamp on to another docket, nodded to the next man, turned the file round so that he could sign, and whispered to Foster: 'Piss off, mate. Can't you see I'm busy?'

The supervisor stood for a few seconds, stunned. It took him a couple of splutters before he could put words together sensibly. Then he said: 'Right, that's it. In twenty-four years you're the most insubordinate box clerk ever to work here. You're going on to an adverse report.'

Before he had time to hump off I turned my back to the queue, put my elbows on the desk and said: 'Who the hell's gates do you think you're talking to, you self-important, puffed up, bloody pigeon. Don't use words like insubordinate to me. I've just had six years of that kind of bullshit. Wipe your arse with your adverse report. And another thing, stand to attention when you're addressing an officer.'

I was smiling when I turned back to the two dozen unemployed lined up in front of me. So were they. Clearly they had heard every word. As Foster strode away muttering, one of them cheered, then another, and finally, the whole bloody queue broke into applause. 'That's great,' I said to the two nearest, 'if I ever stood a chance of keeping the job it's up the chute now.' So when this brought more cheering and handclapping, I surrendered to the inevitable, and, standing back, took my bow.

Just before lunch the phone rang. It was Alma. 'I've been ringing you for two days,' she said. 'Where have you been? I haven't heard a thing from you since Monday night. My God, talk about a letdown! We were so close, too. Could you not have let me know what you were doing? I cried in bed last night. Did you expect me to go to that woman's house looking for you? Are you trying to make little of me? What's wrong? Is this what I can expect, all over me the one day and then disappearing out of sight . . . ' It was exploding all around my head like eighty millimetre flak.

'I'm all right,' I said wearily, 'I was on the beer, that's all. I'll see you tonight. Meet me at the . . . um . . . Star and Garter lounge, eight o'clock, all right? Don't worry, love.'

'I don't know whether I'll be there or not, so I don't.'

'I'll have to go now, love. Bye bye.' I hung up. Bloody women.

More women. One more, at any rate. I landed home to find that Dicky was entertaining the Doctor and the Lawyer, and there was nothing wrong with that, but we had all just finished eating a fish supper apiece, with good thick wallops of buttered bread and cups of strong tea, when the door was knocked. There was Annie Longley, standing, hand-wringing, as if she was Lillian Gish in one of her evil landlord sketches. She looked at the assembled company and asked me if she could speak to me privately, but that only made the others lead forward and earwig more intently, and there was nothing I could do about it.

'It's Dicky's flat,' I told Annie, apologetically.

'No it's not,' Dicky butted in, 'it's half yours, Hughie. We're mates, me and him,' he explained to Annie, but the three of them watched closely as she took a chair and I slewed mine round from the table to face her.

She looked on edge. Her face carried only a dust of powder, she had thrown a heavy woollen cardigan over her shoulders and knotted a headscarf under her chin, she wore scuffed shoes and there was actually a sag in one of her stockings. This woman had so much trouble that she was wearing its uniform.

'I'm really in a mess, Hugh,' she said. She stopped, shook her head, her eyes began to fill.

I could play the thick-wit no longer. 'Come on down to the door, you can tell me there.' I shrugged into my jacket, stood back to let her out, and closed the door on three pairs of bright, inquisitive eyes.

She let out a sigh that seemed to come straight from the heart. 'When I spoke to you that last time I meant to ask you for more, but when it came to the bit I couldn't do it.'

So she'd been taking it easy on me. Any more of this and I'd begin to feel in her debt. I said: 'Look, you can forget about that other money. Scrub it. I didn't expect it back. Take it as a wedding present. I can't do any more.'

She was worrying as much as ever, chewing the inside of her lip. My offer wasn't good news. It wasn't even news. She'd never intended to repay the forty quid anyway. 'I'm in real trouble for a hundred and fifty pounds. Real trouble. I'm nearly crazy.' I sucked in my breath, and she nodded: 'I know, it's bad, isn't it?'

I shook my head. 'I can't help you any more. I'm sorry.' She was looking down at the ground. 'Look, I'll give you another fifty. Then tell John the truth. Tell him you've spent the other hundred. It'll be all right – '

'He'd call everything off. You don't know him. He hates debt,' she broke in. She'd dropped the fancy accent; the vowels were being flattened like potato farls under a rolling pin. 'I'm in real trouble.' She called it reel.

I reached into my pocket, took my cheque book out and wrote one for fifty. 'That's the best I can do, Annie. I can't just give away a couple of hundred.'

She took the cheque, folded it, put it in a blouse pocket. A tiny nod of the head was the only thanks I got. Then she walked away.

NINETEEN

AT MORNING BREAK O'HARE issued a word of caution: 'That Foster's out to get you, Hughie. He's put you on report. Take it easy.'

But my mind by this time was made up. 'Jack, just take a look at me. Do I look like a civil servant? I'm going to pack this job.'

He grabbed me by the shoulder. 'Hold on, Hughie. It's not all like this. Down here in the buroo is the salt mines of the Ministry of Labour. There are offices up in the Parliament Buildings at Stormont where you'll be able to use your brains, and be treated with some courtesy. This is a rough dive. It's because there are so many out of work. There are men out there signing on who would pull the head off you if they thought they'd get away with it. That turns the staff rough. That's how the Fosters of this place are produced. Take it easy.'

I shook my head. 'I think you've got it the wrong way round and that's the trouble. It's the staff who've made the unemployed the way they are. In fact, maybe it's one of the things that's wrong with the whole bloody community. When I was growing up we hated the cops and they hated us, but it doesn't take a genius to work out who started it. It was the cops who had the power.'

'You're getting into politics now, Hughie, when you talk about the community, and I could show you who started it in Ulster.'

'Well don't. You'd blind me with science. But before we go, could you do me a favour? Could you wise me up on Labour Control?'

'Certainly. Call upstairs, Room 26, first chance you get.'

Our Bill was on one of his stealthy runs into town. Apprentices apparently found it easier than most to sneak away from the shipyard and spend time in the centre of Belfast. He called to see me just before lunch time and we went across the road to the pub together. 'John has failed the written exam for the job,' he said. I whistled tunelessly.

'I also had Annie Longley call on me,' I told him. 'One way and another, they're not off to a very bright start. She's a hundred quid down on the till takings.'

'Well, I've just left the house; she came in while I was there and she was full of plans, getting ready to go out and do all the things for the wedding,' he said, 'and she looked cheerful enough to me, all talk about the wedding breakfast, the guests, the honeymoon. She seems to have got dough from somewhere.'

I shrugged. Maybe the talk about needing another hundred was the come-on. For all I knew, it might have been only the fifty she'd needed from the start.

'I suppose she's got her arm into you good and proper,' Bill said.

'Never mind that.' I studied him closely. 'What about you? Have you got your life mapped out, all right? What are you going to do with yourself when you're a fitter, with your time all served. Have you thought about it? God knows, you're the last chance for the family to make its mark.'

The poor kid had nobody now to advise him, or to give him a bit of affection, with Mother gone, and nobody in the house with the time or inclination to talk to him.

'I've made my mind up, all right,' he said, 'I'm going to go to sea as a ship's engineer. That's an officer's job. That'll be two officers in the family.' He sat, embarrassed at what he was going to say; then he went ahead and said it: 'This family has made its mark, Hugh. An awful lot of people joined up in our district, but you're the only pilot. That kind of a mark would do me.'

'If you get cheesed off, don't forget – I'm only across the road. I should have told you this long ago. Step over any time.'

'What about Dicky and those other ones?' Clearly he couldn't make head nor tail of any of the other three.

'They're only characters,' I told him, 'they're easy to get on with, once you come to understand that. They don't actually have likes or dislikes. They just want to be near each other, that's all. They don't mean either to harm you or to do you any favours. If you were to walk in when I wasn't there,

144

they wouldn't mind. You're my brother and they're not about to put you through an entrance exam. Only one thing' – I held up a warning hand – 'don't give the Doctor or the Lawyer any money. They'll tap you, but just say: "Sure where would I get it?" and they'll leave you in peace. It's your place now as well as mine, OK?'

Bill sipped his orange juice. 'OK,' he said, so I went back to the buroo, leaving him sitting with his shoulders back and a smile on his face broader than Oliver Hardy's arse.

During a slack spell in the afternoon I went upstairs to Room 26. It was a fair-sized place, with all sorts of vacancy notices and posters around the walls. Building tradesmen and their labourers were needed across the water to build what were becoming known as New Towns for people bombed out by the blitz; ex-RAF men with air-traffic control, airfield fire-fighting, and luggage-handling experience were being sought for the new air terminal just opened at Heathrow; the Admiralty wanted radio operators; stock controllers were required in the Middle East. There was even a recruiting poster for the Palestine Police. Up at the counter O'Hare was talking to a customer. 'You'll be all right there, Davy,' he was saying, 'it's steady work, a small engineering outfit. You'll be doing the stores, looking after parts, that kind of thing.' He wrote something on a brown card and handed it to the claimant. Then they shook hands and the man walked away.

'It's all in the handshake,' I said. O'Hare gave me the look he had by this time reserved for me: a grin that brought me half into his confidence and a narrowing of the eyes that kept me half out. 'We try to put the right sort into the right jobs,' he said.

'What about the wrong sort, do they get the wrong jobs?'

'You know what they're like: as soon as one gets into a half decent job he's speaking up for more and if you weren't careful they'd have all the good jobs.'

We went over and sat down at his desk. 'I'm in line for promotion, Hughie,' he said, searching for his tobacco pouch.

'To what kind of rank?' I asked. I knew nothing about the rank structure.

'Senior clerk. Do you know this, Hughie, there's men of our age here who'd be content to go no higher than senior clerk in the ministry for the rest of their days.'

'Oh, you don't need to tell me that. I suppose Foster's one.'

'No, in fact he's not. Foster's an established clerk. And he's delighted to be one. That's as far as he's going and he thinks it's plenty, with the pension and everything. Senior clerk would take me over Foster's head.'

'Jack O'Hare, Senior Clerk JP,' I said, 'and by the way, I've got ideas for another Unionist article and a trade-union one.'

'What's the Unionist one?' he asked.

I'd lied about having a trade-union idea, and I'd lifted the Unionist one from a discussion I'd overheard in the tea room. 'D'you see housing?' I said. 'It's important to keep communities together. Don't let all this talk about better houses for heroes to live in lead to the break-up of communities. Don't shift the people – fix their houses if they need it and keep them where they are.'

'I can get you the figures for houses wrecked in the blitz, Hughie. And I can get you stuff on the way they're thinking of dealing with it across the water.' He sat for a bit, thinking. 'Let Ulster stick to Ulster's ways, that kind of thing?'

I changed a wince into a cough: 'Dead on, Jack.'

'Now, I have a brother, as I was telling you, Jack.' I dropped my voice: 'He's a good guy. He has failed the entrance exam for a job. He's one of those people you mentioned who'd have been happy to be a senior clerk here, but there's no chance of that now. He's getting married in a couple of weeks. Could you do anything for him?' I added mischievously: 'He's the right sort.'

O'Hare was staring into the bowl of his pipe. 'I saw that kid brother of yours over in the pub today. How's he getting on in the yard?'

I was a fraction slow in answering; the guy seemed to know everything about everybody. 'Pretty good. It's a pity of him, with nobody at home to fuss over him. John and his woman have their own problems. Great kid, though – I'm dying about him.'

'You would have been away when he got that apprenticeship.'

'I was, out in Italy, at the heel end of my flying.'

O'Hare had the pipe going nicely. He sucked, and blew; when he exhaled there was a tiny sound, pizzum, pizzum. 'That was because of your father. It was your father got him in.'

I laughed. 'How could he? He was dead . . . ' Then I stopped. O'Hare was giving me his long meaningful look. 'You mean, because of the way he died?' I asked. Jack O'Hare was nodding. I wasn't sure what he meant. 'Bill getting that job makes us all right, is that it?'

He made no sign, just sat puffing, pizzum, pizzum. Then he began to tap the burning tobacco into his ashtray. 'I'll see to John, Hughie, don't worry,' he said.

We were OK people. The Reillys were the Right Sort.

TWENTY

IN THE STAR AND GARTER that evening Alma was wearing a brown, fine woollen dress that buttoned up to her neck, and a heavy, darker brown, winter coat with a deep, fold-down collar and long lapels. A light dusting of snow had fallen and in the streets outside the puddles were covered with a thin skim of black mush. Women who could afford them were wearing bootees, and a few women with boyfriends or brothers in the RAF were warm and comfortable in flying boots. Alma wore the cold-weather gear of the kitchen-house belt – ordinary shoes with short woollen socks. Cold and anxiety showed in her pinched face. We were sitting in an almost empty bar and between us there wasn't even the two and a half volts needed to light the bulb in a pea lamp.

'That was awful, the way you just disappeared.' She was holding her sherry, turning the glass, her finger on the rim.

I was feeling brassed off to the teeth. 'Look, love' – I reached over and took her hand – 'will you for Christ's sake stop using the word awful? It wasn't awful, whatever it is that's bothering you, it might have been thoughtless, or discourteous, or even bloody selfish, I wouldn't know, but it wasn't awful.' I felt a real bastard, when it came out.

Alma took her hands away from mine. She put them in her lap. 'I know I'm not very smart' – her head lifted and she met my eyes – 'but there's no need to make little of me.'

I lowered half of my Jameson. 'I shouldn't have made love to you the other night,' I said. I was hoping to hell she wasn't going to cry. I was going to bring it all to an end between us. 'Alma, two nights ago we were very close. You were right when you said it today on the phone. But here's the difference between us: since then I've had a thousand different thoughts in my head and I've done a score of different things, while you've only had one thought, and that's about us, you and me.' She didn't answer; she sipped her drink. 'I am not going to take up an open relationship with you,' I said, 'and if I promised you that I would, I'm going back on it now. I'm in no position to tie myself to you, and that's it.'

'I suppose it's that woman.'

I laughed. 'The day after we made love I told Mary about it, and I left her. I've been living with Dicky on the Duncairn Gardens since.'

'Well, if you've left her, why can't we stay together?' Her voice had picked up. She'd just heard the worst news and the best news of the week.

'We can stay together if you like, but I'm not going to make it official. I had intended to, but now I've changed my mind.'

'Was it the way I was today, on the phone?'

'Yep.' It was a word of Mary's. 'Yep, it was. It certainly was.'

'But I was annoyed because you just vanished. If I'd known you'd left . . . that woman . . . I wouldn't have been like that.'

I took her hands again. 'I'm no good to any woman, Alma. I'm married to the bottle, anyway. I've got a drink problem as big as the Cave Hill.' I shrugged: 'I'm not worth a tuppenny frig.'

Alma had made up her mind to fight her corner. She was sitting up, her eyes were alive again. She picked up her glass and emptied it of sherry. 'Don't say that about yourself, Hughie Reilly, don't. You're just after fighting in the war. I wouldn't expect you to be like anybody else. You're not the same. You haven't been ever since you came home. I saw it in your eyes even before the trouble started. My daddy says it's the same as shell shock.'

I stared. Then I laughed. I couldn't help it. I remembered the wild-eyed, shouting men from the First War who'd roamed the streets of Belfast when I was a kid, shaking their fists at the sky, yelling at ghosts that only they could see, holding their hands to their ears to shut out noises that nobody else could hear. 'Shell shock, is it?' It started a fit of giggling in me. After some moments' concern, Alma first smiled, then she laughed, too. 'Well, I still think so,' she said.

'Open your coat, for Jaze sake,' I said, 'let me see your figure.' I reached over, but she was already loosening up. 'Come on and we'll get a taxi to the Margrave. I want to make love. It's the shell shock.'

150

She relaxed, and smiled. She was lovely again. 'You're awful,' she said.

We went out into the chill of the night and Alma took my arm, hugging up to me. We reached Royal Avenue. It was too cold to stand still, so I led Alma away from the city centre, back the way we came, keeping an eye for a taxi. When we were opposite the Grand Central Hotel I saw one drawing up, so, dragging Alma by the hand, I ran across the road. As the car stopped I went round to the driver. 'Can you take two fares?' I began. Then I saw his passengers, preparing to get out. One was an American officer, but it was his companion I was staring at. I ran back on to the pavement and offered my arm. 'Well, I never,' I said. Mary Waugh was wearing snug-fitting, Russian-style boots. As she pulled herself up on my arm with one foot on the pavement and one still inside the taxi the hem of her dress slid back, showing plenty of sheer stocking above the slanted tops of the boots. She kept holding my arm as she steadied herself, then she let go. 'How are you, Mary?' I looked down into her blue eyes and smiled. Her cheeks were pink, but it was from the cold air. She was self-possessed as she smiled back at me.

The officer was standing politely, a short distance away. I saw on the shoulder of his greatcoat the silver eagle of a full colonel. He was good-looking, tall, keen in the eye, with hair just beginning to silver. I gave him a smile too. 'We are old friends,' I explained.

Mary turned and the officer came to her. 'This is Hugh Reilly; he's a writer,' she said. The officer nodded to me. He wore the caution of the soldier in a foreign place. Then Mary turned to Alma, behind me.

I'd completely forgotten about her. 'This is Alma Conway,' I said. Mary gave her a nod that wasn't friendly;

the American said: 'Pleased to meet you, ma'am', and Alma murmured 'How do you do', only to him.

'Well, that was a nice surprise,' I said. 'Bye bye, Mary.'

She still had the smile for me. 'Bye bye, Hugh,' she said.

'Goodbye, sir,' the American half bowed to us, the doorman pulled the heavy door open, and they went into the hotel.

'Hey, do you want this taxi?' the driver called.

'Yeah, sure,' I said. Then I turned to Alma: 'Did you hear? Mary Waugh said I was a writer. "This is Hugh Reilly; he's a writer." Did you hear her?' I stood, eleven stone of beaming smile. Then I held the door open and stood back. But instead of climbing in she pulled away. I heard muffled crying, then, suddenly, she turned and ran towards Castle Junction.

'I think you've had it for tonight, mate,' the driver said.

'Take me to Duncairn Gardens,' I said resignedly.

I found Dicky with the Doctor and the Lawyer in Jimmy McGrane's. They moved over to make room for me.

'We were just discussing sex when you came in,' the Lawyer said.

'That's what I thought I was going to discuss earlier,' I said, 'but I ended up talking to myself. I met Mary Waugh and I told her I'd finished with Alma. Then I met Alma to tell her we were finished, but then I thought it might do no harm if we had one last fling. On the way to the fling we ran into Mary, and whatever hell way I said hello to Mary it annoyed Alma. She ran off and left me, so here I am, Alma's gone and Mary thinks I'm a liar. So talk about sex if you like, but don't expect any contribution from me. I've finished with it.'

'We're going down to Pottinger's Entry,' the Lawyer said, 'there's an obliging lady lives there.'

They went off to Pottinger's Entry and I went back to the flat. I had the housing piece for O'Hare to do, and there was something else in my head, something that might do for the paper. I took a carry-out of stout with me and from nine o'clock until the headcases came back at half one in the morning I sat huddled over the writing pad in contentment, glad to be doing something that wasn't going to end up in crying.

When the three musketeers came in, Dicky sat down at the table in high spirits. He pulled a paper bag from his pocket and emptied the contents out as the other two watched. He had spilled three decks of cards on to the table. 'Now look' – Dicky's eyes were sleepy with the drink and the words were slithering out – 'these decks are still sealed up, right?' So they were, each in its tightly gummed paper wrapping. 'Now, I'm going to break the seal on that one, OK?' He ripped the paper, broke out the brand-new cards. 'Wait till you see; just you wait.' He shuffled the cards, tried a split riffle and made a balls of it, watched as I shuffled and reshuffled until the suits and values were well and truly mixed. 'Right, oul mate Hughie, now deal me and you a hand of poker.' I dealt five cards each as the Doctor and the Lawyer bent over to watch.

I had a parcel of scrap.

'Hold your hand up: study it,' Dicky said. I fanned them. Dicky's eyes, with difficulty, focused on the cards. 'It's not worth the dirt between your toes,' he announced. He told me the value of four of the cards, accurately. 'The best you could have is two trays,' he said.

I showed him: 'I don't even have that.' I was impressed.

The Lawyer wanted to try it, and Dicky repeated the trick, then he did the same with the Doctor.

'How the hell are you doing it?' we wanted to know.

'Take the cards and study them, go on,' he said. He opened a bottle of stout against the edge of the table and he drank as I studied the backs of the cards, centimetre by centimetre. It was doubtful if the other two could see the pattern on the cards at all, but they, too, were going through the motions. I shook my head. Dicky smiled, swaying. 'Have you ever met Aggie Mateer?' he said. I shook my head. 'Well, we did, tonight. Aggie Mateer has the key to her oul woman's shop in Skipper Street, and what do you think, but doesn't her oul woman sell cards.' He reached over, tried to punch me playfully on the chin and missed.

'As soon as Dicky heard that Aggie's mother had a wee shop, the first question he asked her was if the shop sold cards. He's cute, this wee man,' the Lawyer said.

'Mind you, I was no good with Aggie.' Dicky looked forlorn, then he cheered up. 'But she likes me.'

'She likes him,' the Lawyer said.

'Goes the bundle on him' – the Doctor nodded agreement – 'more so than us. Most surprising.'

'Her brother died out there, probably in Changi. He was a regular soldier.' Dicky's eyes were needing matchsticks. 'While I was steaming the packs open, marking all these decks, and putting the wrappers on them again, I was telling her about the prison camp, about following the Japs to pick up their butts, about the awful Chinese fags, about the itchy balls complaint, and then all the ones that were dying in Roberts Hospital, from dyse . . . dyset . . . the shits.' With this his eyes closed and he fell asleep.

'Aggie Mateer was all over him,' the Doctor said. 'The two of them were sitting with their heads together all evening and you want to hear some of the things he was telling her.

There were these Sikh soldiers who deserted to the Japs after Singapore fell and they were real bastards. D'you know what the POWs did to them when the war ended? They shoved them head first into the bore holes that they used for latrines. Isn't it a delightful story? When Aggie Mateer heard that, she insisted on taking Dicky to bed. Said it was on the house. Said it was the least she could do for a war hero. That was after me and the Lawyer had been to bed with her. When they came out we were kidding her and asking if he was any better than us.'

Then the Lawyer broke in. 'Know what Aggie said? She said that it was a complete relief to go to bed with somebody who didn't want to do anything except hug her and give her a kiss. I think she's in love.'

Bill was spending time in the flat. He even brought his mate and deadly rival Tommy Boyd with him a couple of times. They were fascinated by the circus troupe that I was a part of. The antics and strokes of the other three had both kids spellbound.

'Are you a real doctor?' Bill wanted to know.

'I'll tell you how real I am,' the Doctor told him. 'Drop your trousers and show me your whanger and I'll tell you what age you are by the number of wrinkles in your clinkers.'

Once, when the Doctor came in from a day on the knocker, he threw his little case at Bill, who caught it on his lap. 'You can keep the contents,' said the Doctor wearily, 'I'm sick trying to shift them.'

Bill opened the case; inside were a dozen five-packs of Durex. Our poor kid thanked him, opened a pack, took a single frenchy out, and opened that. His expression when he saw it had the rest of us chuckling.

'Have you ever seen one before?' the Lawyer asked.

Bill shook his head: 'I've heard tell of them, that's all.' He sat, examining the product. 'Do you sell these?' he asked the Doctor.

'No,' the Lawyer chipped in, 'your man's a mannequin in the Durex factory; he gets to keep a few in the line of duty.'

One day Bill had news for me. 'The wedding's in two days, Wednesday. Annie Longley's paid all the bills. I heard John telling the aunts.'

'All's well that ends well,' I said.

'And John's got a smashing job through the buroo. Steward in a golf club, with Annie working there too, and a flat as well.'

I could only stare. O'Hare was awesome.

Next day John appeared on the other side of the counter, wearing his Steward of the Turf Club outfit.

'Hello,' I said, thinking I might as well.

'I'll be sarning off,' he announced.

I took out his file. 'Sarn here,' I said.

'I'm taking up a post' – he was enjoying himself – 'and it'll be a relief to get away from this place.' He looked around with distaste at the queues, at the burly messenger at the door, who held the claimants back by brute force, at the white-tiled walls, at the whole scene. Then he turned on his heel and walked away, and, so help me Christ, he was swinging a blackthorn stick. Today he was a retired colonel of the Inniskilling Fusiliers.

TWENTY-ONE

———————

I WAS WAKENED BY a woman's voice. Bending over me was somebody with orange hair, make-up on her cheeks that looked like distemper on a wall, and thick lipstick, smeared and smudged all around her mouth. 'Do you want a cup of tea, Shooie?' She was holding a steaming mug in her hand. After blinking and sitting up, I saw a big woman, with a lumberjack's shoulders and a bust that could have milk-fed fully grown gorillas. She spoke again – by the sound of her she was smoking fifty a day. 'Are you all right, Shooie?'

I smacked and swallowed a few times, and tried to take her in. She was wearing a man's pullover, a skirt that could have done as the curtain for the Empire Theatre, and about size twelve men's boots. 'I'll bet you an even fiver,' I croaked, 'that you're Aggie Mateer.'

She beamed and it was like the face of the Black Mountain splitting open. 'Sure I know that,' she said. 'Are you getting up?' She laid the tea on the floor alongside my mattress, pulled a butter box close and planted herself on it.

'Are you visiting?' I asked, trying the tea.

'More like moved in.'

As a piece of news, it meant nothing to me. If she'd told me that Belfast Celtic football team had moved in along with her it still wouldn't have stirred my interest.

I stood up. I was wearing only a shirt. It was a short shirt. Aggie sat looking me over, critically. 'That one's seen some action,' she said.

'Being a Carmelite,' I said, 'you would know.'

Aggie stood up laughing. 'We're all going out for a mouthful; are you coming?'

'Well, you've wakened me up, so I might as well.'

We all went out, and I soon found out why Aggie's lipstick was running over. She and Dicky were kissing on average every three minutes.

'Why don't you take him on your knee?' I remarked in McGlade's bar in Donegall Street.

'You mind your own business,' she said. 'He's my wee Dicky, aren't you, dote?' She put her hand down on to him: 'He's my wee Dicky, he's got a smashing wee miniature dicky and I love him.' She said minotaur for miniature.

We tore into bowls of broth and dark, grainy bread. The Doctor spooned a piece of meat out of his bowl; he examined it. 'When that was alive it was pulling a bread cart,' he said.

'Nothing wrong with horse meat,' I said, 'I had it in England. Bury it in broth, well boiled, and it's just the job.'

'Do you know this?' Aggie said, 'I never ate as well in my life as I did during the war. For dear sake, some of the soldiers were paying me in steak and eggs, KO'd out of the cookhouse.'

'Rationing was the best thing that could have happened.' The Doctor was wearing his professional look. 'The poor people got a balanced diet for the first time in their lives, and I would say that things like rickets and bone malformation have dropped dramatically.'

The talk came around to clothes. Neither the Lawyer nor the Doctor had anything left of the clothing coupons issued by the government. The Lawyer was complaining: 'I don't think they give us enough coupons. After all, we have to live. How do they expect us to get through in these times with such a miserable clothes ration?'

This puzzled me. 'I would have thought that the food coupons were more important than clothing coupons,' I said.

'Don't be bloody stupid,' the Lawyer said, 'you need your food coupons to live, but you can sell your clothing coupons for drink.'

I nodded. I'd raised a silly point. 'Mind you,' I said, 'I can see a difference in people's dress since before the war, especially the ex-servicemen. Those demob civvy clothes they give us are far better than the ones we joined up in.'

Dicky joined in. 'When I was at school I used to hate the clothes I wore. My oul fella, stingy oul bastard, made me wear things until I was busting out of them. My bollocks were slaughtering me.' Aggie kissed him fondly.

'You know, we two professional men were lucky there,' the Lawyer observed, owlishly, 'we came from comfortable homes. We had good food, civilised surroundings, and decent clothes.'

The Doctor assented gravely: 'We had nice clothes, it's true, true.'

'That's more than you've fucking got now,' shouted Dicky, pointing to the glad-ragged duo, and he, Aggie and I roared and hooted with laughter.

'What are you laughing at?' the Doctor said to Aggie. 'Sure you look like a refugee from a bloody jumble sale, Primo Carnera's twin sister.'

Aggie put out a hand and restrained Dicky. 'Don't duffy him up on my account, sweetheart,' she said, 'let him slabber away there, sure anybody that needs to have the soles of his feet tickled before he can get a stand-on deserves nothing but sympathy.'

The Doctor stood up, his face red with anger. 'That's unethical,' he shouted to Aggie. 'What goes on when a man climbs into the pit with a brass nail is as sacred as the confessional. Call yourself a pro? You're a disgrace to your profession, madam.'

Aggie landed him back on to his seat with one casual swat. 'For some reason I hate to be called madam,' she said, 'it makes me feel cheap. Call me Aggie or I'll flatten your nose for you.'

We bevvied away in McGlade's as the afternoon wore on. Round about four o'clock somebody suggested going to a pub on Royal Avenue where there was a talking parrot.

'They say if you hold something blue in front of it, it says eff the King, and if it's green you're holding it says eff the Pope,' Dicky said.

'Well then, let's go,' Aggie shouted, and the five of us trooped out of McGlade's into Donegall Street. The Doctor started singing 'The Ball of Kirriemuir', and we all joined in:

> The doctor's daughter she was there,
> She wasna very weel,
> She had tae make her water
> In the middle o' a reel . . .

We were in full song as we reached the Metropole Hotel. A wedding party was coming out. The wedding car was at the door, the bride was in her going-away suit, a tiny knot of people were throwing confetti and rice. The groom ran out behind the bride. The noise of our singing rose above the cries of the wedding guests, and both bride and groom looked over as we came up to their car. I met our John's unbelieving eyes, and Annie Longley's, and our Bill's and the uncles' and aunts'.

And Alma Conway was there, to the side of the group. I began to act drunker than I was, when I saw her. She was wearing a powder blue dress, and long, deep blue gloves, and she was carrying a floppy hat in her hand. I tried to read the expression on her face: whatever it was, it certainly wasn't pleasure, and concern wouldn't have been the right name for it either. It wasn't hard to see how John felt, though.

'You're looking lovely,' Aggie said, and Annie Reilly, as she now was, drew away as Dicky and Aggie both made to hug her.

'Ah,' said the Lawyer, whose fly was gaping wide, 'a wedding. Every good wish, my dears.'

I went over to Alma as the newly-weds were getting into the car. 'You look nice,' I said. She was watching me warily.

She moved away from me and closer to her mother and father, who were throwing confetti over the departing couple.

Dicky was ushering Aggie, the Doctor and the Lawyer away. I put on the Stan Laurel look of the daft drunk, treated Alma to an exaggerated, apologetic shrug, and I followed Dicky and the others, as the wedding car started up and John and Annie set off for their honeymoon.

In the pub with the parrot I threw drink into myself like a docker broaching a whiskey cargo, and we laughed till the tears came to our eyes when it effed the King and then the Pope. We sang songs, old and new, peacetime and wartime, and drunk as I was, I was surprised when Aggie started to sing 'That Lovely Weekend', with her lipstick smeared and drink running down her chin. Her voice was clear and strong and the whole bar had fallen silent by the time she reached the verse where the soldier's leave was over:

> You had to go, time was so short,
> We both had so much to say,
> Your kit to be packed, the train to be caught,
> Sorry I cried, but I just felt that way . . .

She stopped suddenly and we all watched as her face crumpled and she began to cry. Dicky put his arms around her. I watched them, and then I felt a crying jag start up in me, too. I went out into the gents, locked myself in the one cubicle, sat down, and let it run its course. I thought about Mary Waugh.

When I ran out of reasons to feel sorry for myself, I pulled myself together and went back into the bar, where the Doctor was holding his doings, looking down at it, and singing:

162

You are my tart's delight,
And where you are
She longs to be.

I didn't remember getting back to the flat but when I carried my cup of tea to the table next morning, with the others still snoring, I found two notes on the table, written by myself:

Dear Alma, I'm sorry if I let you down today. That's me. It's a good thing you've caught me on. You looked so nice. Now here is something important: go to Corporation Street Labour Exchange, ask for Jack O'Hare, tell him you're my cousin. He'll fix you up with a job. Good luck, Hugh.

The other one went:

Dear Jack, I am not going back. Hope everything goes well with the union venture. My cousin, Alma Conway, will be calling to see you. Hope you can help her. She is due a good turn and this would be your last and biggest favour to me. Thank you for everything. Hugh Reilly.

Amazingly, both notes were written firmly and cleanly. I got out two envelopes, addressed them, threw on my coat, and went across Duncairn Gardens to the post office and posted them. Going back to the flat, I shivered, ran my hand over the stubble on my chin, wondered where I was heading, and then stopped thinking about it. I had the price of a drink and I had uncritical company, so fuck every other consideration.

I made myself some toast when I got back and sat down to the lightest of breakfasts. I'd bought the paper but I wasn't in a reading mood. After a bit, Dicky ambled in, scratching himself. He poured a cup of tea, sat opposite me and opened the paper.

'The Dan Byrne case is on the front page,' he said, sitting up. 'Your man'll be packing his wee bag soon, the one with the straps and the rope and the white cap.'

'Who's that, love?' Aggie, the only one of us who was not, by now, expert in the technique of judicial hanging, had come in wearing only a slip. She'd washed off her make-up before going to bed, and in the raw state her features didn't look too bad at all.

'I'm talking about Pierrepoint,' Dicky explained.

'I've seen him in the Opera House,' Aggie said, lifting the teapot, 'he's a magician, isn't he?'

'He's a fucking magician, all right,' Dicky said, 'he makes people disappear.'

'I know, and he makes water scoot out of their heads.'

'I don't know about that, but I'll bet you a fiver he makes water scoot out of other parts of them.'

'Aggie, dear,' I said, patiently, 'Dicky's talking about Albert Pierrepoint, the public executioner.'

She looked impressed; her eyes rested on Dicky with pride.

The Doctor had joined us. 'Hey, maybe this Pierrepoint thing could help Dicky to perform. It might get rid of his importance,' he said.

'Christ, I never thought of that, Aggie,' Dicky said. 'What about it if you were to be condemned to die and I was Pierrepoint? I could come up behind you, tie your hands, tie your feet, throw you on the bed . . . '

'Amend that,' the Lawyer shouted, 'the woman hasn't been born who could give birth to the man who could throw

Aggie Mateer on to a bed. You'll have to jump into bed, Aggie.'

'I'll jump into bed, you jump on top of me, and we'll see how it goes.' Aggie's eyes were shining. 'I hope it works, Dicky. But not too often, mind. About once every six months. I've had enough of that. In fact, maybe just on your birthday.' They cuddled their way into the bedroom.

I was reading the paper. It was the *Irish News*, read by Catholics mainly, except for dog-racing Protestants. 'They're very upset about this case in the *Irish News*,' I said.

'It's because he's a Taig, that guy Byrne, that's why they're getting so excited,' the Doctor said.

I looked around in alarm.

'What's the matter?' the Doctor asked.

'I hope the Lawyer here's not a Catholic.' I had dropped my voice, in the Northern Irish way, on mention of the subject.

The Lawyer burst out laughing. 'Tell him who's the only Taig here,' he said.

'I am' – the Doctor spread his arms – 'and if I can't mention Taigs I would like to know who can.'

We heard Aggie and Dicky at it in the bedroom.

'It's all right,' Dicky was saying, 'it'll all be over in a second. I'll just put you on the trap, shove this hood over your head, leap to the handle, pull it, and that's your lot. You're in the hands of an expert.

'All right, Mister Pierrepoint, I'll let you hang me, then. Will I jump on to the bed now, love? Are you not going to take your clothes off?'

I went over and closed the door as delicately as I could. Fifteen minutes later they came out. They saw our expectant eyes. Aggie shook her head. 'No good.' She turned and kissed Dicky. 'But mind you, he was excited. I've never seen him that excited.'

'I think we're on to something,' Dicky said.

TWENTY-TWO

T HAT EVENING, AFTER A subdued session in Jimmy McGrane's pub, the Lawyer and the Doctor took themselves off down town to look in on the start of a darts tournament in one of the clubs. It seemed that the Lawyer was a decent thrower, something that had the Doctor and the rest of us baffled, considering the tremble he had after a beer-up. 'Good dart throwing brings drink as its reward,' the Lawyer explained, 'that helps to banish the shakes.'

Dicky was sitting fiddling with the cards, the places were all set for the poker game, when there was the sound of a step outside, the door was pushed open, and Leo Grogan came in. I looked at him, deadeyed, and his glance returned the sentiment with interest. Bucksie followed, and I gave him the same welcome. Bob Mills, a cheerful local grocer, fond of a bet, arrived, then came a wasted-looking man called Gerry something, from the Falls Road, and Geordie McMinn, a small-time bookie. Dicky's marking of the cards caused me a spasm, but he wasn't playing, just dealing, taking a shilling a pot plus tips, collecting his money in a cup. A kettle simmered on the stove, Guinness was stacked in a corner, with five bottles of cheap wine, and Aggie went around and took contributions towards the cost of it all, plus fish supper money. Then the game began.

Aggie was sitting beside Dicky. 'Do we have to stick looking at her?' Leo Grogan asked, jabbing a finger in Aggie's direction.

'What the hell's gates is wrong with you?' Aggie's dander was up. Dicky, recognising the priority of the visitors, squeezed her arm, and made shushing noises. Aggie sat tight, defiantly.

I read the paper. The game went on, talk was low and continuous. Dicky was dealing, shuffling, watching the money drop, calling each player's liability when credit bids were made against high-value notes. I got down to the detail of the Dan Byrne murder case.

'In a navy blue suit, and wearing his wartime merchant navy badge in his lapel, Daniel Byrne, the man accused of killing his wife, Teresa Byrne, in their home at Shipbuoy Street, heard his Counsel, Mr D.C. Bogue, KC, address the jury.

'Byrne had served throughout the war, surviving two torpedo attacks. He married Teresa in October 1945, and she persuaded him to give up the sea. Byrne had taken a job as a casual docker; he was unhappy with the conditions of this work, his wife would not agree to his going back to his job as a bosun in the merchant navy, Byrne had taken to heavy drinking, leading to debt problems, and the cumulative effect of this had brought relations between man and wife to a low point.

'On the evening of the killing, Byrne was bringing a day's earnings home, knowing that there was a threat of eviction if rent arrears were not paid, at least in part. On the way, he called into Mulgrew's public house on York Street, for just one drink. Unfortunately a celebration of some kind was going on, and the accused was the recipient of a good deal of free drink.

'By the time he left he was extremely inebriated. In addition, he had spent his day's pay. Upon arrival at his house a row developed between the accused and his wife. Accused will tell the jury in evidence that Teresa Byrne lunged at him with a kitchen knife, in the heat of a struggle. It was whilst trying to take the knife from her that the blade penetrated Teresa Byrne's chest, and this was the wound from which she died.'

I put the paper down. Poor bugger. I'd started it off with my bloody antics, buying liquor all around the bar.

It was time to get the fish suppers out. Aggie carried them from the stove. She held Leo Grogan's from a height and dropped them in front of him, scattering his notes and coins. I opened mine. The paper was baked on to the fish and chips, but that was no more than we were all used to. Aggie handed out the tea, mostly in milk bottles. I laid my bottle beside me, closed my eyes, and listened to the card talk. The one named Gerry had dropped out, and Dicky wanted his place.

'Balls,' Bucksie growled, 'you're not on. You've only got the couple of quid that's in that cup. Sit there and deal, before I take your few bob and shove them down your throat.'

I went over to the table, put my hand into my jacket pocket and brought out some notes, about fifteen quid. I tossed it on to the table in front of Dicky, and waited for Bucksie's response.

He turned and looked up at me. The pupils of his pig eyes actually seemed to be pulsing with rage. 'What the frig's it got to do with you?' he said as he watched Dicky scoop up the notes gleefully.

I looked at Bob Mills and the penny bookie, and ignored Grogan. 'OK with you?' I asked.

They nodded warily, watching Bucksie.

The big minder got part way up from his chair. 'See you, big mouth,' he said, 'you watch it.'

'Talking about big mouth,' I said, nice and quietly, 'when you open that hippopotamus mouth of yours all we can see is half-chewed fish and chips. For Christ's sake swallow the stuff before you try to talk.'

'If I was you,' Grogan said to me, 'I would mind my lip. I want to play poker, but it'll not worry me too much if Bucksie there takes you out first.'

'How are you at handling yourself, Grogan?' Aggie put in. 'Does big balls here do the fighting for you?'

Grogan was sorting his money out, putting the coins in neat piles; he ignored Aggie.

'Are we all right, then?' Dicky was shuffling the cards. He placed the deck in front of me. 'Want to do dealer, Hughie?'

I sat in the empty seat, took the cards, shuffled them, held them out for Bucksie, jumping mad as a hornet, to cut. Then we started to play. Right from that first hand, Dicky began to win. His first victim was Bob Mills. I pressed my foot on Bob's. He'd already dropped about fifty quid, mostly to Bucksie, so, on receiving my signal, he stood, stretched. 'That's me out. Good night, all.'

As he left the Doctor and the Lawyer came in, grabbed a bottle of wine from the stock and disappeared into the bedroom.

In less than ten minutes the bookie followed Bob Mills, after losing in a head to head with Dicky, beaten by a pair of sevens. So far, neither Grogan nor Bucksie had been dealt useful hands, but they'd noted the run of things and were watching Dicky closely.

By now I wasn't worrying a ferret's fart about the cards being marked. There was a feeling growing in me that I knew very well. The sooner Bucksie tackled Dicky the quicker I could get at him.

Aggie, not knowing what was going on, began to clap her hands and kiss Dicky. 'You're a great poker player, darling,' she kept saying, but soon after, she must have received some kind of warning from Dicky, because she, too, rose and went into the bedroom. Soon I had to go and close the bedroom door, as her wine-induced snores joined the hallelujah chorus of the Lawyer and the Doctor. That left just the four of us. In another ten minutes Dicky had cleaned Bucksie. Halfway through the bidding on his hand the minder snapped his fingers to Leo Grogan who passed some notes to him. Dicky lifted the money and threw it back to Grogan: 'Your mate can't borrow to bet, he can only borrow to see.'

'Up yours,' Grogan snapped. 'Go ahead and bet, Bucksie.'

'That's the rule of poker,' Dicky said, 'it's the rule everywhere.'

All of a sudden Bucksie threw his cards in. 'There's something funny going on here,' he said. He took a deep breath, his nostrils flared, and he spread his hands out on the table.

'If you can't take it you shouldn't dish it out,' I said. 'There was nothing wrong with this school when you were skinning Gerry and Bob Mills, now all of a sudden there's something funny going on.'

'Wait a wee minute,' Dicky said, 'houl your horses, lads. I'll open a new deck. It might change your luck, Leo. Just the two of us, eh?'

With the opening of the new pack I reached over and relieved Dicky of the fifteen quid I'd loaned him. Smiling at Bucksie, I dealt the cards for the final showdown. 'I hope wee Dicky takes you to the frigging cleaners here, Grogan,' I said in a conversational tone.

Bucksie's chair barked as he shoved it back, but Grogan held a hand out. 'There'll be plenty of time for what you want to do, Bucksie, but before you do it, I want to tell the shithouse clerk here a thing that I want him to know. But play cards, eh?'

'Sure,' Dicky said. He was sitting, fancying himself as Humphrey Bogart, with the smoke blinding him in the one eye. I dealt Grogan two pair and Dicky, with one pair, packed without betting. I dealt Grogan an ace high and Dicky went for him with two jacks. Finally they got into a betting situation, with a prile each, of which Dicky's was the better. The final bid from Grogan was Dicky's thirty quid and another thirty over it.

Dicky said: 'It's always a pleasure to see a good loser: your thirty and how's about half a hundred more, to keep the pot warm?'

Grogan sat, studied, thought, looked at Dicky, then at me. 'I'll see you,' he said.

Dicky fanned his hand on the table.

'By the waters of Babylon, there we sat down and wept,' I said, as Grogan flung his cards down and sat back. 'The last time you played with Dicky you seemed to think he wasn't in your league,' I said as I gathered up the cards. 'Well, what do you think about him now?' I was watching Bucksie out of the corner of my eye as we all rose.

'Do you want a bottle before you go?' Dicky went to the crate in the corner. He knocked the tops off three and gave us one each. Bucksie put the bottle to his mouth and, with one foot on the chair, let the stout run straight down his throat without a swallow, but Grogan was sitting, eyeing me. 'What have you got against me, you, Shakespeare, hey?' His lips had gone tight with the loss of the last hand and they hadn't filled out again.

'I don't dislike you,' I told him, 'there's room for everything in this world. I'm just protecting this wee man. It just happens to be an unexpected pleasure when looking after Dicky means fucking you two up.'

Bucksie growled into action. 'You must be good. You've got plenty of brass neck. But I can't see it. You look easy enough to me, you long drink of pump water. I could take you aisy.'

Start now, I was singing inside. I knew there was going to be a move, but I thought it would come from Bucksie, aimed at me. So that's what I was watching for. Grogan was to my right, in front of the fireplace, facing me. Bucksie was to my left, with his back to the door. Dicky was at the other side of the table, murmuring to himself, almost crooning, counting his money, and there must have been a couple of hundred quid of it.

When the action came, it was the last thing I was ready for. Suddenly Grogan snatched up the poker from the side of the hearth. It was long and it was heavy, three quarters of an inch the whole way down its two and a half foot length. I jumped back, out of range of the swing, but, missing me, he let Dicky have it right across the side of the head. The little man slumped over the table at once. By the sound of the crack his jaw was broken. Grogan held the poker high, watching me.

'You've killed him,' I whispered. I was sure of it. Dicky's breathing had become half snore, half snuffle. His face had swollen already. The swelling had ballooned out all the wrinkles he'd brought back from the Far East. He was unrecognisable.

I had no weapon. I was watching Bucksie and Grogan.

'You stupid bastard,' Grogan said, 'you and that fucking halfwit there. You give me the shits, with your fancy talk.' His voice rose. 'Well here's something for you to talk fancy about, I'll tell you a story for the paper, you bigheaded get.'

'Take it easy,' I said, putting a whine into my voice. It had worked before, gained me time in bar fights. It worked now. Contempt showed on both their faces. 'That guy needs help.' I nodded in Dicky's direction, almost bleating. Bucksie was scared, seeing Dicky's condition. He'd had enough. He had no plans for further action, but Grogan was riding high.

'You listen, Reilly. I want you to listen, right?' he said.

'What?' My voice was dull, deferential.

'That fucking hoity-toity sister-in-law of yours, Annie, that was Annie Longley, right?' I tightened up, had to work to hide it. 'Well, Mister Bighead, we've both been there, Bucksie and me both, so up yours, you fancy-talking fuckpot.

174

She fell behind and she paid up, OK?' He rammed the poker into my stomach. I almost grabbed it, but decided to wait for a better chance. 'She was lovely and juicy, wasn't she, Bucksie? It's been a long time since I've enjoyed anything as much. And I'll tell you better – she still owes me. We've still to collect, haven't we, Bucksie?'

But the minder wasn't in a gloating mood. Dicky was still making half-smothered noises; every now and then a breath would end on a deep moan.

'I was the first one there, shithead. D'ye hear that?' Grogan's voice was high, almost a shriek. His lips were wide in a sneer, and drink had reddened his eyes. 'All night I've been dying to see your face when I told you.'

I stood, let my shoulders slump. I lifted both hands to shoulder level, as if in surrender. Grogan nodded, satisfied. He had already lowered the poker. He glanced at Bucksie, who turned to the door. Grogan left the poker down on the hearth. He began to button his coat.

I reached him in two steps. The stone mantelpiece hit him just underneath the shoulders as I chested him. I stood back, as he arched from the pain, and I let him have a short chop to the point. Then I gave him a left, and as he slumped down and into the fireplace I heard the door open and Bucksie run on to the landing and down the stairs.

I lifted the poker, moved Grogan's head to a suitable lie with my foot. I stood back, measured the shot, waggled for aim, and let him have it with my full weight, exactly across the spot where he'd struck Dicky. Then I did it again. It felt like smashing into plywood, with a cork lining. I threw the poker down and went into the bedroom.

The Doctor and the Lawyer and Aggie were out like lights. I hauled Aggie up and shook her awake. 'Go and help

Dicky,' I said. 'He needs an ambulance. I'll ring for it, you just look to him.'

At the door I turned: 'Grogan's out there too. He's only for the bin.'

TWENTY-THREE

T HE PRISON GOVERNOR'S NAME was McMahon; he was an ex-army major. He was embarrassed when he visited me: 'Everything all right, Reilly?' He was red-faced, sandy-haired, with the usual army small scrubby moustache. His accent was County Antrim, with an English overlay. 'If there's anything . . . ' he would say, and he'd wait, search for more to say, fail to find it, then turn abruptly and leave.

The screws told me that this wasn't typical, that it was only with me that he was uncomfortable. 'It's because you're an ex-officer,' one screw said. 'I heard him remark when he read your file that it was an odd thing for an officer to do, and odd company for an officer to keep.'

'I suppose he's right, at that,' I replied.

As the screws went back to the crossword puzzle in *Reynolds News* I lay stretched out on the bed with my hands behind my head and went back to thinking about our John. In the weeks that had passed since I'd rung for an ambulance for Dicky and walked into York Street RUC barrack, I'd thought about John an awful lot. It was natural, I suppose. He was at the heart of all this.

I was lying in remand, on a murder charge, in Crumlin Road jail. I had killed a man. There was a chance that I'd have killed him for what he'd done to Dicky; there was a better chance that he'd have been killed for what he'd done to Annie; but my view of it was that I had killed Leo Grogan for what he had done to my brother John. Once I'd grown used to doing without the bottle, and started to think, I thought, more than anything else, about John. I'd never wanted to go against him, I never had, in fact, yet he actually seemed to hate me. Well, now, of course, there'd be no seeming about it – he really must hate me. It wasn't as if I'd always been a pain in the clinkers to him. There'd been a time when he was an OK brother, not close, in the way that Bill and I became, but all right, as good as the next. I liked him then, and he liked me. That was until I took the beating over him at school. It all started when John mitched to be with Ellie Coates.

Ellie was thirteen and she lived like a gypsy in a rough-and-ready shanty down at the Corporation tip head at Alec's Bank. She had turned up there from nowhere. She and her father, whose lungs were in tatters from mustard gas, rummaged amongst the rubbish for damaged fruit and saleable household items. We kids used to go down to Alec's Bank for a swim at the lip of the harbour entrance, that's how we got to know her. She wasn't fat, wasn't thin, was friendly with us when her old man wasn't around. One day when our John was in the water in his drawers, Ellie took her dress off and joined him.

I could see, from the distance I was ordered to keep, that they were showing each other their parts. She had breasts like mandarin oranges but our John had developed. I knew that because he slept in the front attic with me. I heard John ask her where her oul fella was. 'Oh, he's in the hospital again,' she said, 'he won't be out for a couple of weeks.'

They went, the two of them, to the hut. I hung around waiting, and when John came out he told me that he was going to mitch school to be with Ellie Coates all day.

Next day, a Monday, I told Morton, John's teacher, that my brother wasn't well. It was tonsillitis, I said, and it was looking as if it would last. Meanwhile, John nearly wrecked his own plan because he came home looking very clean.

'You look as if you've been swimming,' Mother said.

I covered up for him because he was so slow. 'A whole lot of them were acting the goat, ducking their heads in the sink after the science lesson,' I told her.

Two days later there was another enquiry from Morton and I said that things were getting worse.

'Any word of you coming back to school?' I asked John. He shook his head.

Next Monday the question came again, and the next Wednesday. By that time I was shaking my head and saying that we were all getting worried about John. And on the Friday morning he was nabbed.

A neighbour man who had a plot down at Alec's Bank had spotted John, luckily on his own at the time, rifling amongst the rubbish, and he sent him home and ordered him to own up. The first I knew of it was when Topcliffe, the headmaster, called me out to the door, where Mother was holding John by the arm. Naturally, Ellie Coates wasn't mentioned. The funny thing was that both Topcliffe and my mother agreed that John should receive only light punishment. Topcliffe said: 'That's the longest any boy has ever mitched, we'll need to be careful that he doesn't become a delinquent. As for you' – he grabbed me by the ear – 'this would not have been possible if you hadn't lied consistently throughout. You are going to be severely punished for this.'

'Yes,' Mother said, 'go ahead. He's more to blame than John.' Which I thought was a good one. John got the girl and I got the hiding. This must have been the caning that so impressed Mary Waugh. My crime was announced and I was beaten in front of the whole school, except the infant classes. During the course of this ordeal something happened to me that was to last for the rest of my life. I saw the whole thing as an act of loyalty to a brother, but my defiant expression sent Topcliffe astray in the head. 'Are you sorry?' he would thunder. 'No!' I would shout back. 'Then I'll beat you until you are!' Miss Davis, my own teacher, had to jump in at the end and protect me, or Topcliffe would have landed me in hospital.

After that I was never afraid to stand up to authority. I never trusted people in high places. I never took bullshit from anybody again, and I set about learning to protect myself. By contrast, John was taken by the hand; Mother bought him new clothes, she encouraged him to take an interest in church affairs, he became a youth leader, and took to playing badminton, which we all called babbington. I was quite proud of him, but he certainly wasn't proud of me.

When I was at myself again after the beating, I went down to Alec's Bank. Ellie Coates had gone. The hut was derelict, empty, except for a huge rat, which ran over my foot on its way out.

We weren't at odds as we grew to manhood, but we had little in common. In his new life John chose friends from the semi-detached belt, people who called dances hops, had parents who could afford to pay their way through grammar school, worked at clerical jobs, wore good suits to work. John wouldn't let any of his car-driving friends pick him up at our house, he'd meet them along the way. When the night's jollying was over, he'd ask them to leave him off on the Duncairn Gardens, where the houses were half as big again as ours. And he got himself a job in J.P. Corry's, the timber yard; an office job, working for buttons. But when Dad died, he was head of the house.

It was then that the real rows began between us. I wasn't the earning type. I was sacked out of half a dozen message-boy jobs for daydreaming and mixing up customers' orders. I was usually lying on the sofa reading when he came in from work, and he would kick me off it. I suppose, to be fair, the first umbrage came because he could have been doing with a hand in keeping the house running, but as we grew older things got worse. In time he got over the shame of living in a kitchen house and allowed his friends to call, but when they did I wasn't just idle and scruffy, I used to tap them for cigarettes.

When the war had been on for four months or so John joined up and so did I. He and his friends joined the same regiment, I went into the RAF. He would rather I'd stayed at home and looked after Mother and Bill.

TWENTY-FOUR

T HERE WAS NO ARGUMENT about it, the first few days of my jailing were pure hell. Not because of the grilling, or the police activity; indeed, the bluebottles were quite friendly, it was a nice case as far as they were concerned, neat and tidy, no great trouble. They were good to me, sat talking in my cell about things outside of my crime, about their own problems, about what they called the real villains, as if I wasn't one. No, the first days of the brig were days that I didn't want to remember, as the poison left by ultra-heavy drinking fought and resisted its voiding. Hallucinations and Holy Christ wake-ups, soaked in boozer's sweat, when I got sleep at all, left me twitching worse than a third tour air-gunner. They thought at first that it was post-arrest shock, but a police doctor tumbled and I got vitamin injections up the chuff and psychiatric counselling, and, gradually, things got better.

That racking fortnight stood to me. When I came out of it, and became fit again, I was better able to face my short future. The tales told by Dicky about Pierrepoint also helped; at least I wasn't left wondering about what was going to happen when the time came. I knew every detail. At the end, when the screw would offer me a drink, I'd know that the hangman was in the cell behind me, and that if I put my hand out for the whiskey, he would grab it, and the other one, and pinion them. So, making it easy for him, I'd put my hands in Pierrepoint's. Not that he'd appreciate it. Any man who could eat bacon and eggs and then straight off do a hanging couldn't be called perceptive.

There were riots by loyalists outside the jail. I hadn't heard any of the noise from my remand room in the hospital wing, but I was allowed to read the papers. Dan Byrne's plea of manslaughter had been accepted by the State. He'd been sentenced to ten years. On the other hand, my case looked an open and shut neck job. But Leo Grogan had been a Catholic. The loyalists weren't on for a Protestant suffering death just for killing a Catholic, especially after Byrne had escaped the rope. Outside of political murder, Northern Ireland was relatively free of serious crime. The last man to be executed at Crumlin Road jail had been Lieutenant Tom Williams, Acting OC of C Company, 1st Battalion, Belfast Brigade of the Irish Republican Army, for shooting dead an RUC sergeant in September 1942, three years and a half ago, and that was exactly how the loyalists of Belfast expected the gallows to be used. In fact, five others had been reprieved, in the Williams case, a decision which extreme loyalists regarded as lack of moral fibre on the part of the authorities.

The various court appearances leading to my trial, due in the Belfast City Commission in three days, were no mental ordeals to me. I just sat and didn't look around, didn't look anywhere, except straight ahead at the bench or at my hands.

Apart from my solicitor, a guy of my own age called Jack Rice, and my barrister, a walking icicle called Lagrue, I wanted to see very few visitors. Dicky could see me any time he wanted, and Aggie Mateer did bring him, but the blow from Grogan had finished off what the RAF and the Japs had started. Dicky was smiling and retarded. He didn't know where I was, never mind why I was there.

'I wanted to see you about something,' he said, the first time.

'What was that, Dicky?' I asked.

He sat, smiling his Fred Astaire smile. 'Ah, what's this it was? Right. Here's what. You're my mate, aren't you?'

'I'm your mate, all right, best mate, Dicky.'

He nodded, still smiling.

Aggie was looking after him in the flat. 'Here, Hughie, he's awful fond of you,' she said.

'You're a good woman, Aggie. Are you OK for a bob or two?'

She gave me an old-fashioned look, and I had to smile.

The Lawyer and the Doctor had been to see me as well.

'Aggie threw us out of the flat,' the Doctor told me.

'Well, I suppose she wants to clear the decks to look after Dicky,' I said.

'Sure we could look after him, too.'

184

'Well, why don't you prove it to her? Give her some dough. Let her see you mean it.'

'Give her dough? Is your head cut?'

'We need every halfpenny we can get for the drink,' the Lawyer added, 'I don't suppose you're anyway well fixed yourself?'

This incensed the screw who stood near me. 'Christ, that's the worst I've ever heard. The man's in for murder and you're tapping him. Have you no skin on your face?'

The Lawyer beckoned to him. 'Tell me, my man,' he said, in his best courtroom voice, 'have you ever heard the one about the explorer in Africa who was shown two prized delicacies by the chief of a cannibal tribe: they were the brains of two victims. "One ounce of lawyer's brain, here," the chief explained, "and it cost me two goats. And that other one is an ounce of Crumlin jail screws' brains, and it cost me fifty goats." '

The screw looked pleased.

'And when the explorer enquired as to why there was such a difference in price, the cannibal said: "Have you any idea how many Crumlin jail screws it takes to make up an ounce of brains?" '

I wrote no letters from the jail, and I asked Aggie to let everybody know that I didn't want to receive any. I didn't want to know who amongst my friends had been to my preliminary hearings and I didn't look to see when I was brought into the dock. Bill came to see me in prison but the visit was a disaster. He broke down and had to get up and leave after about three minutes.

I was tempted, over and over again, to let Mary Waugh know how I felt about her. I wrote letters to her, all right, but they ended screwed up on the floor. I wasn't allowed to

185

tear them up: it appeared that the prison doctor wanted to see my written work. It would probably earn him a Ph.D. one day.

Still, the issue of Alma Conway was settled fairly conclusively. That one was dead, all right. Uncle Sammy asked, through the solicitor, if he might come to see me, and I agreed. What a pleasant, innocent man he was, all round-eyed, looking at the surroundings, and obviously full of concern for me. I think he'd have wanted to see me anyway, for we'd always got on and he'd tried to help in the row between John and me at Mother's wake. But I sensed an equally strong purpose in the way that he brought Alma into the talk, without any encouragement from me.

Alma, he told me, was in a good job, and he supposed that I'd be glad to hear it. She was working as a clerical assistant in the women's buroo in Alfred Street. She'd been desperately upset about my trouble, like all the family, but this fellow she was starting to go out with, an office colleague, was a big help.

To make it easy on Uncle Sammy and his family I explained that I wouldn't be writing to anybody and I didn't want anybody writing to me. I told him, in a man-to-man kind of way, that the hardest part of that was the fact that I would probably never know how Mary Waugh felt about me, and he couldn't keep the relief out of his soft eyes. There'd be no letter from me to Alma.

The screw called Danny was a drinking and gambling man, full of zip one day, biting his nails the next. He had more life in him than the rest of my minders put together. They were regimental, strict, but when Danny got the chance he was fond of registering solidarity with me by letting me

186

know that he was a fiddler, flogging smokes to short-term prisoners who weren't allowed them at all, carrying messages to friends outside, that sort of thing. In fact, of all the screws in the Crum, he was the obvious one for O'Hare to use in order to make contact with me.

Danny was on his own when he said, two days before my trial: 'No matter what happens, keep your chin up, Hugh.' He said this with an odd intensity, and a glance full of meaning.

I stared at him and said: 'They're bringing a man over specially to do that, or didn't you know?'

He laughed, shaking his head in admiration. 'You're a real hoot, Hugh, but anyway' – he lowered his voice – 'O'Hare says to tell you to keep your hopes going. There's a chance, that's all he says, there's a chance.'

I could only blink for a bit. 'What the bloody hell can he know?' I said.

Danny's eyes were on the door, watching for his mate. 'There's holy murder threatened outside over you. The Prods aren't happy. Maybe it's to do with that, I don't know. Don't ask me how O'Hare's mind works, but he's no mug,' he said.

I was angry. 'This is a shit's trick. There's no changing what's for me.' It wasn't fair to lift my hopes, now that I'd worked out a routine, a way of being flip, to cope with doomsday. Suddenly I was in a high state of nerves. This was all bullshit. But still, O'Hare was in the picture, the master fixer. 'Christ, I hope he's right,' I said and began to whistle, then I cut it off, annoyed with myself. It was a bad habit.

'If trouble starts up in the streets, O'Hare's the boy'll use it to help you in some way. He's the most loyal Prod I've ever met, and the craftiest bastard in Belfast,' Danny said.

Smoothly he changed the talk into a joke about an Englishman, a Scotsman and an Irishman, and I heard the sound of his mate's step outside.

I lay on the bed as the two prison officers fixed up the Monopoly board, but no matter how hard I racked my brain I couldn't work out what O'Hare was up to.

TWENTY-FIVE

'T HEY'RE DESPERATE WORKED UP about your man Dan Byrne,' the screw remarked as we sat in the room under the courthouse, 'this place was like Casey's Court last night. They had every Prod hard man in the town lined up opposite the jail gates to show us how they feel.'

'Glad I wasn't there. I suppose it means something to them,' his mate said, 'but they can't change the law. That's up to Stormont.'

'They're beginning to gather out there this morning again' – the first one shook his head as he said it – 'you would need to be blind not to see what they're after – it's the jury they want to get at.'

'Dressed well, that's good, Hughie.' Rice nodded, looking me over, pleased. 'It always helps. You've the RAF tie on too.'

'I didn't know there was a Raff tie till you handed it to me,' I told him.

'Sit up nice, the way you've been doing up to now. If a Crown witness says anything damning, shake your head, as if to yourself, unbelievingly. You're in the papers as an ex-RAF officer, so keep looking like one.'

I had been brought there by way of a tunnel that crossed the Crumlin Road.

'What'll it be like in the court?' I asked Rice.

'You'll see when you're brought up.'

I liked that bit about being brought up. There was a strong dungeon smack about it. Actually, when the time came, the words that were shouted and repeated along the echoing passageways were: 'Send up the prisoner Hugh Reilly.' So the jury was in place, the trial was about to begin, the Belfast City Commission was in session. I was pleading not guilty to murder, and I was being sent up from down below, like one of the Bounty mutineers. So much for the neat clothes and the tie, and the brushed hair. With an introduction like that, not even Laurence Olivier could have made an effective entrance.

With a screw on each side of me, I was led up a dozen steps, there was a sharp turn, another seven steps, and I was behind a four-foot-high oaken partition facing the judge. Remembering the advice of the solicitor, I stood just short of parade attention. I could feel the eyes of everyone in the court drilling into me.

'Are you Hugh Reilly?' a loud voice rang out. The clerk of the court was quite a young man. I looked him in the eye.

For Christ's sake, I told myself, with panic lapping my mind's edges, don't say: 'The very same', or 'That's me'.

'Yes,' I replied, not too loudly, but clearly enough.

'The charge before the court is that you, Hugh Reilly, on the seventeenth day of April in the year nineteen hundred and forty-six, in the county and city of Belfast, murdered Leo Grogan. How do you plead, guilty or not guilty?'

'Not guilty.' According to Rice, I was supposed to add my lord, but balls to him. The judge was a big, round-faced man, in a crimson cape, with a wig that was too small for him. His name was Mr Justice Thomas Quigg – real Dickensian, that. He was looking at me keenly, with open curiosity. This surprised me: OK for the jurors and press and public to gawk at me like a carnival exhibit, but judges saw felons all the time. Maybe it was this guy's first murder case.

I didn't know what the hell kind of an expression was on my face as the screws motioned me to be seated, and the show got on the road. I hoped it was an intelligent, attentive look, sharp, a bit like Stewart Granger as a wronged defend-ant. But more likely I was coming across as a middleweight, down-the-card fighter, during the introductions, making monkey faces with his gumshield.

To my right, the business of swearing the jury began. I had imagined that this would all be over before I arrived. This process took about twenty minutes and helped me to steady myself for the hard times to come, for the swearing-in ceremony by the clerk of the court included, for each juror, the solemn instruction: 'Prisoner, look upon the juror', and 'Juror, look upon the prisoner.' By the time I'd looked upon the fourth juror I'd found a formula: the thing to do was to take an interest; the thing to avoid was to work at taking an interest. It was at this time that I found it was easy to keep from looking at the public gallery.

The judge told the jury that they would be under protective custody for the duration of the trial, he gave them ten minutes in which to go to the jury room and send messages to their homes.

Then the business of the trial proper began. There were to be nine witnesses for the Crown and five for the defence, the case was expected to last for three days.

McAuley, the Attorney-General, was leading for the Crown. He told the jury to set aside any feeling that this was a special case; nothing, other than the cold facts, should influence them. He was tall, not bad-looking, about fifty; he spoke in a plain voice, the vowel sounds surprisingly flat and homely for a King's Counsel.

He told how I had walked into the barrack and given myself up, that there was blood on my clothing at the time of my arrest, and that forensic evidence would show that this blood was of the same group as the victim's. There were fresh abrasions on the knuckles of my right hand consistent with the delivery of a blow or blows. The Crown would produce the only witness of the attack and this witness would testify that the attack was unprovoked.

Now I really was listening: I had no trouble at all in delivering the slight, unbelieving shake of the head, as advised by my solicitor. The tale was that Grogan took the poker in his hand to defend himself after I had struck him on the face. In the ensuing struggle I had wrenched it from him and struck the fatal blow. Probably by accident, in the course of the attack, another person present was struck a blow by the poker and was very badly injured. The Attorney-General went on to talk about fingerprints on the

192

poker, of which one set would be shown to be mine and another the victim's.

Leo Grogan was described, not as a moneylender, but as a financier, a businessman, unmarried. He'd been relaxing, the jury were told, playing cards in a flat which the prisoner shared with others, when the attack occurred.

The Crown would produce evidence that I was a person of unstable temperament, a heavy drinker, who, at the time of the murder, was in danger of losing a good job in the civil service, because of unsatisfactory conduct.

I had to stop myself from nodding agreement with that bit.

It was a funny feeling, though, to hear the facts of the case so neatly upended. And to realise that it didn't really matter about that in the final reckoning, because the Attorney-General could hardly have been faulted in his final words to the jury: 'As this case proceeds I feel sure that you, members of the jury, will agree that what happened in the early hours of April seventeenth was murder, and that there is no other name for it.'

The procession of Crown witnesses began. I tried to follow my solicitor's advice and stay alert, but the courtroom was packed, the air was stale, and, anyway, I didn't want to hear what they were saying in the witness box: I wanted it all to go away, either that or for my case to collapse. I wanted it over with.

Bucksie told a pack of lies, that my attack had been unexpected, that Grogan had lifted a poker in the face of my attack, that I had wrenched the poker from him, swung it, missed, hit Dicky, then struck Grogan and threatened himself, forcing him to flee for his life.

The right time to let your thoughts go for a ramble is when

the talk comes round to Injuries Sustained by the Deceased.

Japonica
Glistens like coral in all of the neighbouring gardens
And today we have Injuries Sustained by the Deceased.

Now the fucking poker was out in the open court. By God they were making good time on this case. It was covered in cellophane and held by a court skivvy. 'Would you examine that poker, please?'

It was carried to the pathologist, who looked more like a joky bus conductor. 'Yes, the injuries sustained by the deceased were consistent with blows from this poker . . . Number of injuries . . . Fractures . . . temporal bone on left side . . . blow delivered . . . angle such . . . fractured also occipital bone . . . damage . . . the parietal and occipital lobes of brain . . . death would have followed in minutes.'

Good.

'Would the blows have had to be delivered with some force?'

'Considerable force.'

'Delivered by a man of some strength, for example?'

'Certainly by someone who was athletic, who knew how to swing the weapon concerned to maximum effect. There was no evidence of injury to the deceased's arm, as in warding off the blow, so one inference is that whoever delivered the blow managed to surprise the deceased completely.'

Or managed to land one on the whiskers and have the bastard halfway to bye byes before swinging with the number three iron.

There were more Crown witnesses, a sergeant of the RUC to confirm that, whilst he was on barrack duty, Hugh Reilly walked in and said: 'My name's Hugh Reilly; you don't know me, but you soon will.' And a sergeant plain-clothes detective to describe how he'd cautioned me, and charged me, and how I'd made no reply when charged. Then the first day was over and I stood up, turned one hundred and eighty degrees, and went down the steps.

As I rose I'd caught a glance out of the corner of my eye at the jury. It was time for them to go, too, but, to a man, they chose to sit and look upon the prisoner. All the way down the dark of the stairway, and across the tunnel, with its bare electric bulbs, their gaping stayed with me, running down my face, like raven's shit.

TWENTY-SIX

D OWN BELOW, BEFORE THEY moved me back through the tunnel, Rice told me that the case would take three days. 'Lagrue isn't happy that you're refusing to testify, says it cuts his options and I agree, Hugh.' He looked worried. 'You've a good appearance, you'd make an effective witness. You don't mumble and you don't say too much. As we've told you so often, the position you're in is tantamount to a plea of guilty. It's a pity you won't open out, get into detail about the incident.'

Incident was a great word. Breaking Leo Grogan's head was an incident. In 1941 every German bomb that burst open a Belfast slum and creamed its occupants was an incident.

'If the Crown were to go for you, we think you could handle it. There's goodwill for returned fliers. If you don't testify it will make things very difficult.' He went on to remind me that the defence could show that Grogan kept some very shady company. 'But if we trot that out without putting you in the box to back it up, the Crown will make out that we're simply blackening a man's name when he can't answer for himself.'

I shook my head. If I were to testify, I might, under stress of questioning, maybe as a reflex reply to a prosecution taunt, tell the truth about Grogan and Annie Longley. Nobody knew about it except Annie, Bucksie and me, and it would stay that way. Neither Bucksie nor Annie would talk about it, and, by God, none of the other women that Grogan had raped would rush to say so.

And, anyway, even if the defence were to show that my attack on Grogan was a reaction to his treatment of Annie, it would make no difference. Knocking him cold in the old-fashioned way with one to the button would have been enough; to put him asleep, then crack his skull with a poker was plain murder. I would still walk the chalk, and the lives of Annie and John would have been ruined for good.

The prison doctor was called. He said that, in all essential regards, I was sane, that I was rational, and that in his professional opinion at the time of commission of the crime, I was fully aware of what I was doing. I knew what this was all about: the chance of a plea of insanity on my part looked to have been blocked off.

Then up stepped the psychiatrist for the defence. I'd had several talks with him in jail, a nice little man, pleasant, hadn't seemed the least bit probing. Rice had explained to me that he would be talking about my flying record. Right enough, he'd shown a lot of interest in that. 'Give me an example: run through an operation,' he'd asked.

Well, Ploesti was a good one. We were supposed to spend lots of effort into putting the Americano Romano oil refinery in harm's way. It was to the west of Ploesti town, twenty miles north of Bucharest. Trouble was, every mile in the Balkans, on the ground, in the coastal waters, and in the air, was murder mile. The airspace was defended by night-fighters in numbers, as well as the most stinking anti-aircraft fire outside of Berlin. When a night-fighter arrived, it arrived very quickly. Your leg gets itchy, you reach down to scratch it and find that you can't, because you've got no arm, it's been blown away by twenty millimetre. And the whole air force knew, if the public didn't, that all that stuff by the bomb-aimer – 'Left left, right a bit, skipper' – went up the chute when you were coned in three bright blue lights. 'Hold it another ten seconds,' the bomb-aimer shouts, and the pilot tells him: 'Drop the bastards now and my arse on another ten seconds.' Dives get you out of cones, but you're not three seconds into a dive when four lanes of twenty millimetre slice through the cold light stretching ahead of the aircraft.

What you do then is try to make a bomber into a Spitfire, throw it about while steepening the dive, and you scream 'Fighter! Fighter!' as the four Brownings in the rear turret begin to bellow. Suddenly you see the fucker swimming into view, ahead and above. He's lost you, but he hasn't missed altogether, because there's no answer from the rear turret, and there's a smell of burning coming through from the back.

Over to starboard, a little red rose grows in the sky, and it grows until it becomes a burning bush, dropping.

Somebody's trying to dive a fire out, but suddenly a jet of flaming fuel trails out from the heart of the thing and then there's the explosion. The brain holds a snapshot, as an aeroplane breaks up. You see the mainplanes leave the fuselage, the gap between the wings and the root ends left behind, then it all disintegrates into flaming falling debris. But, anyway, it's not you.

The navigator puts your fire out with a hand-held extinguisher, so it wasn't all that much of a fire. But the rear turret's gone, and the gunner's not there. Well, he's there, but only part of him. A shell went off inside him. His head has fallen between his feet. The rigger doesn't half flake out when he sees it. Talk about flake out.

'Did you discuss the death of Mister Grogan with the accused?' Lagrue asked the psychiatrist.

'I did. He refused to talk about the incident.'

'What conclusion did you draw from the prisoner's lack of co-operation in this matter?'

'That, mentally, he was almost untouched by the incident.'

'Would you link this with any part of his background?'

'It is possible that it arises from his wartime experiences. He was pilot of a bomber, operating against heavily defended targets in central Europe. On many of these operations his aircraft sustained attack; he had crew members killed twice and two others badly wounded. It was common in the war to see air crews distance themselves in their minds from violent situations. And, of course, as the First World War showed, continuous exposure to danger blunts the senses in violent situations, even away from battle.'

'Would you describe this distancing as a consequence of battle fatigue?'

'Yes.'

'Of course,' the Attorney-General said when Lagrue had finished, 'another name for it would be callousness.'

'What you term callousness tends to be a comprehensive feature of a person's nature. Insensitivity is usually displayed to other people's feelings generally. I found no indication of this condition where the accused was concerned. His reactions differed from the normal only in violent situations.'

Beside me, Rice breathed out as if this was going to help. I was buggered if I could see how. My feeling was strengthened when Aggie Mateer was brought to the witness box to describe the scene in the room after I'd woken her up.

Aggie, dressed in an imitation leopardskin coat, with the paint thick on her face, spoke directly to the judge, turning round to face him with each reply. 'Well, sir, your lordship, I was right and tired and I'd had a right few liquors, and I couldn't tell you what went on before Hughie Reilly there woke me up, but I'll tell you one thing, if Hughie did this, well then, that bloody bastard Grogan deserved it.' Her voice rose as she talked over the judge's cautions. 'No woman that borrowed money from him was safe. He took it out of any woman that fell behind with the payments. Sure everybody in the city of Belfast knew him for it.' Now she was shouting over the objections of the Crown, as well. 'What the hell's gates do you think he kept a sofa in his office for, the dirty baste.'

She stopped. I breathed a sigh of relief as the judge threatened her with jail if she didn't restrict herself to evidence that was relevant to the case. For a while I'd thought that Aggie knew about Annie's loan from Grogan.

'How do you make your living, Miss Mateer?' the Attorney-General asked.

'I'm on the game, your lordship. Why, what has that got to do with anything?'

Everybody in the court was laughing, except the judge, Rice, Lagrue and me.

The hearing was adjourned at five o'clock. The jury would hear closing arguments and the judge's summing-up and go into their huddle the next afternoon. I watched them file out. Not one of them looked at me. I'd read somewhere that, when the accused was doomed, the jury didn't look at him as they came in with their verdict. This bunch had stopped looking at me before the frigging case was even over.

As I lay in bed that night my thoughts were so scrambled and wild that sleep was a thousand to one shot. In the early hours of the morning, sheer fatigue and wretchedness had weakened my brain cells to the point where I was ready to consider a desperate plan.

At the start of my imprisonment the governor had told me that, if I ever wanted it, I could always have something to help me sleep. I'd refused. There was no point. It wasn't as if I had an appointment or anything, or work to go to. If I couldn't sleep through the night, then I could make it up through the day.

But how about it, my sick brain asked, if I were to begin now, and for all the nights left to me, to ask for the old knock-out drops, then, somehow, save the tablets up, hide them, and take the bloody lot the night before my date with Pierrepoint?

I gave it a whiz. At three in the morning I sat up. 'Could you give me something to put me over?' I asked.

'Certainly.' The screw got up, went out, and came back with a steaming cup of Horlicks.

That straightened my thinking. It also left me whacked for the first part of the last day of the trial, the final submissions and the judge's summing up. Not that any of it made good listening. Lagrue did what he could for me, but had nothing to work on, except the suggestion that Bucksie and Grogan had moved in a moneylending underworld, an argument for caution in accepting any evidence given by Bucksie. But he was still lumbered by the fact of my having given myself up, and, most of all, my refusal to testify.

For McAuley, it was money for nothing. He only had to ask the jury to consider the facts of the case, and to take into account that the defence had been unable to cast doubt on one particle of the evidence given by the only eyewitness.

As far as the summing-up was concerned, it sounded like a recording of the Attorney-General's address to the jury.

At 4.30 p.m. the jury went out. I was taken downstairs to the usual cramped room. The police brought sandwiches and tea for Rice, Lagrue and myself. The other two tucked into theirs with gusto, but my share stayed on the plate, although I needed the tea for my dry mouth.

Suddenly I felt sick, physically. I began to sweat; I knew that I must be pale. I bowed my head and fought it off. I was trembling all over, then the sweating stopped, and I felt cold.

'Are you all right, Hugh?' one of the screws asked.

I breathed in deeply, nodded, and it passed.

'Don't forget, Hugh,' said Rice, with his mouth full of bread and corned beef, 'there's still the appeal, and we have grounds that'll take them by surprise. We'll say no more now. Just keep going the way you've done up to now.'

The cups and plates had only just been taken away when a court official came in, all excited and urgent. 'The jury's back,' he said. They'd only been out thirty-five minutes. Talk about open and shut.

The Clerk of the Crown and Peace asked the foreman of the jury: 'Have you reached a verdict?'

'We have.'

'How do you find the defendant, guilty or not guilty?'

'Guilty.'

All around the court there was a rustling. A kind of sighing filled the room. Underneath me, the lawyers began to tidy their papers. The warders urged me to my feet. For sweet Jesus' own sake hold steady, I thought, you're all right, no sign of nerves, that sickness below settled you. The clerk was asking me if I had anything to say why sentence of death should not be passed on me. I was standing straight. I made no reply.

'Hugh Reilly.' This was the judge. 'You have been found guilty by a jury of your fellow citizens upon convincing evidence of having murdered Leo Grogan on the seventeenth of April last. It was a brutal murder and I endorse the jury's verdict.'

Pretend it's an inspection. Thumbs in line with the seam of the trousers, stare at a point five degrees to the side of his eyes, chin in, chest out . . .

The black square was placed on his head. 'The sentence of the court upon you is that you be taken from this place . . . '

Don't breathe quickly, or it'll start something. That's it.

' . . . and that you there suffer death by hanging, and that your body be afterwards buried within the precincts . . . '

Steady. Steady.

' . . . Lord have mercy on your soul.'

I didn't have to keep it up any longer. With the last words of the sentence I was almost hustled down the stairs. I heard a woman cry out, and a man shouted at the judge: 'You Fenian bastard.' Then I was out of it. There was no need to go on with the pose, but I held it, anyway.

Rice and Lagrue came down. Rice said comforting things, but Lagrue, in a ceremonial kind of way, took my hand in silence and shook it. A screw told me later that this was something that counsel for the defence felt bound to do in murder cases, when it was a hanging match. It was owed to the condemned. A convention. Something that one must do, you know.

TWENTY-SEVEN

'WE'RE APPEALING, OF COURSE, Hugh,' Rice said, before the screws hurried me back through the tunnel to the Crum.

'If you're appealing, it means that the date doesn't apply,' an English warder told me. He meant the date of my execution. I was to learn that the word would never be used in my presence.

I thought that I'd be hurried out of the hospital remand wing into the death cell as soon as I got back. I didn't want to go. I didn't want to move. The room in which I had lived since coming to the Crum was now my home, the most friendly place in the whole jail. In any case, there was a terrible dryness in my mouth. It wouldn't go away. And my thinking processes seemed to have seized up, too. When I was better they could move me.

It got worse when they took my civvy clothes away and made me wear a rough white prison shirt, and trousers made of poor quality cloth. But at least they weren't rushing me to the condemned cell. I was to spend the night in my own familiar room. In the prisoner's clothes that they'd given me, I sat on the edge of the bed, felt for its metal edge, ran my hand along it, like a man patting his much-loved dog. Every few inches, at the tie for the wire cross-piece, I stroked it, leaning along the bed to go from tie to tie, caressing the cold metal.

I let my chin rest on the blanket, even buried my face in it. My stomach felt as if it was supercooled, like the hailstones that are suspended in the cumulonimbus cloud. I plumped the pillow, smoothed it, tidied the blankets and sheet. In the air force, when I was an aircraftman, we'd have a kit inspection every Saturday morning, our kit laid out on the bed, each item in its proper place, and the bedclothes were in tension, without a single ripple or wrinkle. I worked on the bed in my room in the hospital wing, watched in silence by the screws, until I had made of it a bed fit to be inspected by the most finicky of orderly officers, and when I had finished I stood and looked at it, and rubbed my hand with my chin, and I looked at the screws and I said Oh God Jesus Christ, Jesus Holy Jesus.

It was two days before they took me to C Wing, to the condemned cell. I spent them tidying up my room, over and over again. It took the two days, full out, before my mind was in any sort of steady state. It took that long before my tongue came wet again. When I could begin to reason it out, the fact that there was to be an appeal, that my lawyers thought it worthwhile, helped me most of all to face the move to the death cell. At least Pierrepoint wasn't going to come for me on Wednesday the nineteenth of June. There would be a stop to all that and a new date fixed. It would be five weeks before the appeal, and the thing was to happen three clear Sundays after that, so I had eight weeks now, instead of eighteen days.

When the move came I had worked out a trick to get through it. I pretended that it was a posting to a new RAF station. I'd done it so many times, walking into the hut on a new unit, dumping my stuff on the bed, asking the other guys what the place was like, which pubs were the best bets for women, what the grub was like. The RAF was a lonely life sometimes. Just when a man had made friends on the camp and set up connections locally he was posted sometimes hundreds of miles away. After a long train journey, reporting in to the guardroom, learning his hut number, then starting all over again to make friends. So I persuaded myself that this was just another move to another camp.

I had to have something to carry to C Wing, but I had no possessions, none. So, walking between the screws, I carried my slippers. I went through the door and into this big cell, much bigger than the room I'd left. I walked straight over, threw my slippers on to the bed, sat on it, bounced on it, turned to the two screws, threw my arms out, and said: 'What's the grub like around here?' After two days of seeing me silent, sleepless, licking my dry lips, they were so pleased that they both, spontaneously, half-hugged me, as if we were footballers, and I'd scored a winning goal.

This was the way to play it, I thought. It was easier on me. It wasn't long before I was in the same kind of mode that had seen me through the pre-trial times. I'd been in jail three months, after all: I was a twig in the jailhouse stream, or a leaf blown along in the jailhouse wind, or any other frigging metaphor that anybody felt like conjuring up.

For a week or so I had stopped swearing. Inside me, I'd been wondering why there was a kind of rubbing brake-shoe effect on me in those first days in the old DC, as I began to call the death cell, and that was it – there were no oaths to lubricate my language, to make it flow. It was stupid. There was no reason for me to stop effing and blinding, so I went back to it and at once felt better for it.

There was, naturally, a Bible by my bedside. In all the time I'd been in the brig I'd never read it, and, in case there was a chance that I might, I'd given orders from the start that I didn't want any clergy next nor near me. But damn it to hell didn't I lift it after about ten days in the DC, and it fell open at Galations 6.7: 'Be not deceived; God is not mocked: for what-soever a man soweth, that shall he also reap.'

I read it out to the death watch. 'My arse on that for a sentiment,' I said, 'take that and lose it.' But, sheepishly, he told me that the Bible had to stay in the DC, and that was that. So I put it out of sight, under my mattress.

Time went on, and, since the next item on the agenda was the appeal hearing, I forced myself not to think about the land that lay beyond it. But within the range that did exist, one thing was worth thinking about – O'Hare's curious mes-sage, and, in this regard, I was screaming inside for another chance to talk to Danny.

He was on the death watch. There were six warders on shift, two at a time, four on and eight off. Apart from Danny, I called the others by their numbers, starting with One and Two on the twelve to four shift, Three and Danny, who came on at four, and Five and Six, who worked from eight until noon or midnight. Through the days and nights when Danny was on, I found myself almost praying for the chance to talk to him.

It was difficult; even when the screws needed to take a leak they used the pot in the DC, but one day, two weeks after the trial, the chance came. The governor called at seven one evening, shifted from one foot to the other, cleared his throat, asked me if there was anything I wanted, then, as he was leaving, he called Three to the door. 'You wanted to see me?' he said.

'Yes sir,' replied Three, 'but it might be one for the prison board.'

'Well, let's see, tell me about it.' And they moved out of the DC, around the door, and out of sight.

Danny had caught my eye; he was ready.

'Anything from O'Hare?' I asked.

He shook his head. We were both watching the door; we could hear the murmur of conversation from just outside.

'All I know is what he said, to keep your chin up,' he said.

A hundred times I'd tried to work out what O'Hare had in mind, or whether, indeed, he had meant anything by his message, other than to cheer me up. I'd fantasised a Jimmy Cagney scenario, somebody slipping me a gun, shooting my way out, hijacking a car on the Crumlin Road, the Orange Order spiriting me off to Omaha and a new life, running a filling station. Another was the old cyanide capsule trick, to be bitten just as Pierrepoint looked into my eyes, but, in the end, the most I'd hoped for was that he'd arrange for me to have the best legal brain in Ulster for my appeal, some sharpshooter who'd blind the court with science, proving that the murder could only have been committed by a left-handed man. Common sense told me, though, that appeal courts only listened to new arguments, new grounds to reconsider, and there simply weren't any.

But a niggle in my mind, arising from Danny's earlier hint, was reminding me that there was a battleground outside, nationalists and loyalists fighting for control of the Six Counties, loyalists shouting outside the Crumlin Road jail because a Protestant might swing. In that context, all sorts of bending and twisting was possible, and O'Hare was as much at home on that battleground as Montgomery had been at Alamein.

When Three came back he said: 'Know what I was asking the Guv there?' I shook my head. 'I was saying that cells . . . like this . . . ' he paused, delicately, ' . . . should be allowed to have a wireless.'

'Well, my goodness, what a good idea,' I said, and Three blushed.

I still went tight on the visits, although Dicky always had preference. He came to see me, with Aggie to look after him. He seemed better in the mind, although his walk was a bit jerky.

'Ah, Mary gave me a kiss,' he said. His mouth was hanging open all the time now and Aggie would reach over every now and again and wipe the dribble with a hanky. She had him looking nice, in a new navy suit, with a white, open-necked shirt. I complimented Aggie on it. She beamed her pleasure. 'I got the price of that in three nights,' she said, 'a big Canadian aircraft carrier's in. There's eight hundred sailors on it.' She took Dicky's hand.

Dicky was watching her closely. He nodded, almost out of breath with excitement. 'We're going to see him,' he said, 'we're going to see Pierrepoint.'

'Ssshhh,' Aggie said and she looked at me apologetically. 'That's all right,' I told her.

'Will you not be seeing him?' Dicky sat up on his chair, with his arms folded, like a kid on his first day at school.

I heard the screw click his tongue, and I turned and reassured him with a wink. 'Yes, Dicky, I'll be seeing him,' I said. 'And you got a kiss from Mary Waugh?' Just saying her name gave me pleasure, but pleasure was dangerous, it pulled sadness along behind. Dicky nodded again. I glanced at Aggie.

'Mary called, the night your trial ended. That's the first time she's been,' she said.

'Has she been to the court?' I asked.

Aggie shook her head, thank Christ. 'You should have seen the crowds outside our flat,' she said. 'The ones living there are kicking up holy hell, the woman that owns the place wants us to get out, but it doesn't worry me or Dicky.

'Mary sat talking to us for, oh, about two hours. She brought some nice cake and buns and stuff, and a bottle of that rye whisky that the Yanks drink, and we talked and had a wee drink and the time didn't half go in.'

I wanted to ask if she'd mentioned me, but she must have; she was bound to; Jaze sake, I'd just got the works from the judge, hours before. But I waited.

Then Aggie said: 'She cried. Mary cried. I've never in all my life seen Mary Waugh crying. Never in my life. But she cried sore, Hughie, about you.'

'What did she say, when she was crying.'

Aggie didn't answer for a bit. She sat holding Dicky's hand; she was wearing a blue beret, which she'd pushed right to the back of her head as she talked, and she was sitting with her legs wide apart, her skirt hiked up, about half an inch of make-up on her face, a real character. I wasn't expecting a sensible answer to my question, but she said: 'What do you think, Hughie? Are you fucking stupid? The woman's crazy about you.'

TWENTY-EIGHT

TWO OF THE SCREWS were members of Alcoholics Anonymous. Five told me about his drink problem. 'Thanks to my Higher Power, I've arrested it now,' he said, 'I'm doing the Steps.' Then Six chimed in: 'Me too.'

'What steps?'

'The Twelve Steps.'

'What twelve steps?'

They went through them: powerless over alcohol; lives unmanageable; decide to turn to God, etc., etc. Finally, the twelfth step: promise to carry the message of AA to other alcoholics.

I stared. They were looking at me with the sort of shine in their eyes that Four Square Tabernacle evangelists have as they sing on a hot summer's day and wake up everybody on the beach. 'Are you Twelfth Stepping me, for Christ's sake?' I said.

'Well, yes. If anybody had a drink problem you had. Hadn't you?'

I didn't know whether to laugh or cry. 'There's a man coming to Twelfth Step me proper. Have you forgotten that?'

'Who knows what the future holds?'

I waved their offer away, but at the same time it certainly made their watch interesting, since I was tuned in so closely to the drink frequency. Five and Six were real AA converts. The movement had only just reached Belfast, and these two were founder members. They spoke their own quaint language:

'Alcoholism is the only sickness that tells you you haven't got it.'

'One day at a time. Keep it simple. Mind the stinking thinking.'

'You'll keep paying the drink bill long after closing time.'

Without saying anything to the two screws, their long confessions, the testimony of their drinking past, and the relief that this so clearly gave them led me to speculate on the sort of life I might have led outside if only I'd been able to handle the stuff. God, I could have written all day and half of the night, joined a writers' group, a political party. By now I might have read the works of the great writers. In all the time I'd been locked up I'd wanted neither to read nor write, apart from the screwed-up notes to Mary. If the booze and I had only agreed I might by now have written plays, instead of one or two miserable, skimpy articles.

I sat and listened, pretending unconcern, as the two screws happily charged their batteries with AA wisdom. Once, Five actually made me burst out laughing. He was so fired up that, catching my eye, he uttered another of his favourite phrases: 'This, too, shall pass.'

Stupidly I had assumed that I would be in the appeal court for the hearing. There was a new, well-known KC on my side, Butler-Forsythe. He and Rice had explained that the appeal was to be based on grounds concerning some sort of irregularity where the jury was concerned, something about their supervision during the trial. They sounded confident, but I wasn't fooled. Jack Rice was a nice guy, trying to make me feel good; he was too nice, really, to be a criminal lawyer.

'It'll take two days and the appeal judgment will be announced on the third morning,' Butler-Forsythe told me. He was a handsome man, tall, slim, about forty-five, with that slightly effeminate upper-class look that I'd come to know so well in the RAF.

But I wasn't going to get to see the appeal. There wouldn't be any witnesses. It would all be done by legal submissions and arguments, in front of three judges, one of them the Lord Chief Justice. Big stuff.

'And what if we win?' I asked my KC. I'd thought about this. Winning an appeal could mean a retrial, and bollocks to that.

'There's no question of a retrial,' Butler-Forsythe said, 'if we win, you can go home.'

Two and a half days. Sixty hours. It was a long time to sweat. When Rice had been trying to lift my spirits by enthusing about the strength of the appeal grounds, I had said to him morosely, 'I don't know about firm grounds; personally, I would settle right now for touch and go.'

'Oh, we're on the right side of that,' he'd replied.

215

Once, at Foggia, I was relaxing down at the flight, sitting in a deck chair in the afternoon sun, when a Beaufighter joined the circuit. We had a squadron of them on the airfield. Earlier, they'd been practising steep glide approach landings, and often, during these, one of them would touch and go – roll along the runway, open up, and take off straight away. Here was another, I thought, but, instead, this one was in trouble, returning from an operation. It tried the steep approach, all right, but the minute it touched the deck its undercart folded, the Beaufighter skidded for a short distance, then up it went in one tremendous, almighty explosion.

'Christ,' I breathed, as the crash siren went, 'I thought it was only a touch and go.'

'Well, Paddy,' said one of our pilots, 'if that wasn't a touch and go, then what the fuck was it?'

Waiting in the condemned cell, I cursed my brain for thinking that one through without permission.

On the evening of the second day of the appeal Butler-Forsythe and Jack Rice came to see me. Rice was clearly excited, and the barrister, in his controlled way, seemed pleased as well. They explained what was happening, but I couldn't go along with their enthusiasm, flushed and all as Rice seemed to be. Everything seemed to hang on some point of law concerning outings taken by the jury on a couple of evenings during the trial. To me this wasn't exactly the kind of material that made for stage exits from jail, to the accompaniment of cheering loyalists.

The way I saw it, winning the appeal didn't hold out any more for me than the promise of staying alive a few months longer, until another trial could be arranged. No matter what the lawyers said, I still thought that I'd be buried in lime before the autumn leaves began to fall. They left, after urging me to keep my spirits up. It worked to some extent. When they'd gone I thought, well, when all was said and done, all forms of life resisted death to the limit of their strength. It was better to be alive than dead, even in this place.

The fuss started from immediately after lunch the next day. One and Two, most surprisingly, were called out of the DC at one thirty, for some sort of whispered conference. Sitting alone, in the big cell, I closed my eyes tight: the dryness came back into my mouth. They came back, but they were different.

'Has the verdict come in?' I asked. My voice was a croak.

They shook their heads. 'Nothing's settled yet,' One said.

I kept rubbing my chin with my hand. The two screws didn't seem to know how to handle whatever it was they'd been told. They sat, one on each side of the bed, with their legs stretched out, every now and then looking towards the door. I was swallowing and walking up and down the cell, and around and around it. I couldn't sit or lie down. A dozen times I asked them for information, but they shook their heads. Then I heard footsteps outside. They stopped. I thought, sweet Saviour, here it comes.

The governor came through the door. Behind him was the principal prison officer. I was standing by the table. I very nearly held on to it for support. Then I remembered how I'd taken the death sentence in the court. I took a deep breath and waited for it. How was it supposed to go? The Home Secretary sees no reason to change the due course of the law?

But what the hell was I on about? That bit wasn't supposed to happen until the day before the Thing. What was going on? Were they going to do it now?

Danny came in. He was carrying what looked like the washing, in a big brown paper bag. What the frig was happening?

The governor cleared his throat. I held my breath. I could actually feel stress pain in my chest. Everything behind the governor faded, became dark red. I saw his face in the hole that was left. He spoke: 'Reilly . . . '

My eyes closed. There was no way that I could take this calmly.

' . . . The Appeal Court has ordered your immediate release. Your conviction and sentence have been quashed.'

TWENTY-NINE

T HE GOVERNOR WAS BESIDE ME. The others were watching. I held my breath for about five more seconds, then, as I let it out, the backslapping and the hubbub started.

There was a recurring twitch at the side of the governor's mouth. I took this to be a smile. 'You carried yourself throughout with credit, like' – he searched for the words – 'like a commissioned officer.'

'Great show, Hughie,' said One, as Two nodded and beamed.

'Here's your civilian clothes, you can put them on.' Danny was delighted, as he handed over the bag. The shine in his eyes was a million candlepower.

'There is quite a commotion at the gate, Reilly,' the governor said quietly, into my ear, 'I'd advise you to wait for some considerable time. We'll let you out the back way.'

They took me down to the visiting room for ordinary prisoners, and in no time it was filled with warders wanting to congratulate me. One of them told me that he was on gate duty: 'So I couldn't get to talk to you while you were in here, but I'd love to have done. You were number one with all the staff in here, Hughie, but you were more than that with some. Up Ulster, mate, know what I mean?' He winked. I nodded, in a dream.

'You'll be needing a drink,' somebody said.

'And a stiff one too, eh, Hughie?' another voice put in.

The smiles broadened as a bottle was produced: 'Say when.'

I reached out my hand. The tip of my tongue went slowly around my lips. Then, at the back of the little knot of warders, I saw Five and Six. They were happy for me, smiling broadly, like all the others, but there was a different look in their eyes as I took the glass, a resigned look. C'est la vie. They didn't blame me, in the circumstances.

I drew my hand back, and so help me Christ I found that I was clasping it in my other hand, as if to block its way to the bottle and the glass. 'Make it a good strong cup of char,' I said. They were the first words I'd spoken since learning that I was free.

I didn't look to see the reaction of Five and Six. Anyway, I thought, it was nothing to do with them; let's skip it for now and see how we go.

I turned to the governor. 'How did it come about?' I asked.

He drew me a little to one side. 'To be truthful, I don't

know . . . er . . . Hugh. It was something to do with the jury separating one evening, when they were allowed to go out for a drive. First I knew was the instruction from the Appeal Court to release you.'

'Had you any idea about it beforehand?' I asked.

He hesitated. 'Of course, I'd spoken to your people; I knew that they considered themselves to be on strong ground.' He stopped, looked at me. 'If you're wondering why you had to go through that dreadful ordeal without a scrap of comfort, remember that it would have been most injudicious of me, or any of the prison staff to comment on the strength of your appeal. What if we gave you hope, and the appeal was lost?'

I nodded.

Two lived on the Limestone Road, near me. 'Why don't you spend the night in our house?' he suggested, 'there's only me and the wife. There's a whole crowd gathered outside your flat on the Gardens, waiting for you. You don't want that. I'll take the wife out and we'll leave you to meet whoever you like this evening.'

I travelled with him, lying on the back seat of his Morris as it drove out of the back gate into Cliftonpark Avenue and through a crowd that sounded a hundred strong. They were singing and chanting.

'Red white and blue, all the way through,' Two muttered over his shoulder.

As they cried 'Up Ulster!' I lay low on the seat and composed my guest list.

It was a comfortable, wide, double-fronted house, with a small garden, well-kept, and a high hedge. At the door I asked Two for his real name, so that I might greet his wife properly. He told me it was Alec Barry: 'But for Jaze sake don't stop calling me Two. That name's mine in work for life. It's the same with the whole deathwatch. We like it.'

His wife was tall, thin, upright, with keen eyes. Two had let her know I was coming. I wondered how she would greet me. This was my first meeting with the outside world. She put out a hand and I took it. 'You're welcome to stay here,' she said, removing her hand after the briefest of touches. Her manner was formal. Two looked embarrassed, but I was relieved: formal was OK; it was recoil I'd been afraid of.

· We were drinking tea when my barrister and solicitor arrived. Two made them drinks, and he and his warmly-impressed wife left us.

Before the appeal they had explained the grounds to me, but I hadn't been in a listening mood at the time. The way I'd worked it out, counsel and solicitors went in for this kind of talk to comfort the condemned man. Now, they were highly delighted, of course. 'This makes legal history,' Butler-Forsythe told me. 'It'll be one of the most talked-of law reports for years.' They showed me the evening paper.

THREE JUDGES FREE
REILLY

EX-RAF OFFICER RELEASED

In what is thought to be the first ruling of its kind, the appeal of ex-RAF flight lieutenant Hugh Reilly was allowed today by the Ulster Court of Criminal Appeal. The court's judgment was heard by a large crowd in the public gallery; there were also many members of the legal profession in court to hear the historic ruling.

Hugh Reilly's conviction and death sentence for the murder of Belfast moneylender Leo Grogan were quashed. The Lord Chief Justice, Lord Hall, stating that the court had no power to order a retrial, the court ordered the immediate release of Mr Reilly.

JURY SEPARATION

The grounds on which the appeal rested were that the established procedures for the separation of a jury in a murder trial were not followed in this case. The facts, as outlined by Counsel for the Defence, Mr R. Butler-Forsythe, KC, were as follows.

The jurymen were lodged in a small hotel in Carrickfergus. At the end of the first day of the trial they got permission from the judge to go into the town for exercise. This they did, accompanied by a constable.

On the following evening, without permission from the trial judge, seven of the jurors, with a jurykeeper, went out, walked along the shore, and returned to the hotel, one juror stayed in the hotel, watched by a jurykeeper, and the other four, with a jurykeeper, went to Belfast, using the bus provided by the court to convey them to and from the trial. This group drove to Belfast along the Shore Road, turned up past Carnmoney cemetery to the Antrim Road, drove along it, down Duncairn Gardens, past the scene of the crime, to York Road, and returned to Carrickfergus. There they called into a church hall, where a Church Missionary Society exhibition was on display, before returning to their hotel. Again the jurykeeper stated that, although there were members of the public present at the exhibition, there was no contact between them and the jurors.

The trial judge reported to the Appeal Court that he had not been advised of any irregularity on the jury's part during the course of the trial. He had agreed to allow the jury to go out on the evening of the first day of the trial, provided that they would be accompanied by jurykeepers, constables sworn to their duties. No permission was sought or given by the trial judge regarding any outing or bus journey on the second evening, nor was this second outing reported to him subsequently. Beyond this, the judge could add nothing.

The Lord Chief Justice, in his judgment, said that, amongst other things, no judge would have allowed some of the jurors to travel so close to the address where the crime had been committed. He would have arranged for all to go, or none at all, and, in the event that he might have arranged for the whole jury to go to the scene of the crime, it would have been done under proper viewing conditions.

By a most unfortunate sequence of events, arising from he knew not what set of misunderstandings, the proper procedures regarding the separation of juries in cases such as this had been departed from to an extent unknown in past trials. Continuing, the Lord Chief Justice said that, under the law, the separation of a jury was not permitted at any time, in a trial for murder. Extensive search of law reports revealed no record of any trial where deviations from the normal procedure such as had occurred in this case had taken place.

Here the Lord Chief Justice quoted various cases at length, going back as far as the mid-19th century, where the question of unsatisfactory conduct by jurors had arisen. 'The position is that the facts in this present case have had the effect of invalidating the verdict,' the Lord Chief Justice said. 'This court has no power to order a retrial. The conviction, therefore, must be quashed.'

When the announcement was made that Hugh Reilly was to be released, there was some applause from the public gallery, but generally reaction to the decision was confined to earnest, sometimes excited, discussion of the outcome by members of the legal profession present in the court in considerable numbers, including students under training.

LOYALIST DEMONSTRATIONS

A large crowd formed outside the gates of Crumlin prison, in anticipation of Reilly's release. They included many of his neighbours. He was born and brought up in the Duncairn Gardens area. The crowd sang loyalist songs, and displayed loyalist emblems.

Another crowd later gathered outside Reilly's home on Duncairn Gardens, which was also the scene of the crime. Both here and outside the prison, police constables were present, but, although there was some party singing, there were no incidents.

'Did the jurymen and keepers believe that they had the judge's permission to go out that second evening?' I asked.

'It must be assumed that they did,' Butler-Forsythe told me, 'although the Court of Criminal Appeal is concerned only with the effect of the outing on the trial.'

The lawyers stayed long enough to speculate on my future. It made dry listening. 'This will stay with you for the rest of your life,' you understand. You were not proven innocent, but were released on a technicality. It would be my guess that you will find it hard to remain a private person. Your future would be best secured outside Ireland.'

I nodded. Like a light year in distance. It would be no hardship. I hated all of it, loyalism versus the green, white and gold. Dan Byrne had been a Taig; he killed a Taig; I was a Prod who'd killed a Taig; my case was seen against the background of two flags. The real facts of each case were unimportant, World War Two was unimportant, measured against the Irish Question. For Christ's sake the half of my craze for Alma had been because she was Catholic, and what hell sort of society was it that made religion heat up the hormones?

The lawyers left, and Two and his wife returned. 'We're going out, to give you a chance to meet your family and friends,' Two said. 'Give me all the names and addresses, write your messages, I'll get you paper and envelopes.'

I sat down and wrote notes; Two and his wife invited me to use the full facilities of the house and they left. I sat in the quiet house. Outside there was a bus stop. I heard the Cavehill Road bus pull up, the high squeal of the brakes, then the conductor rang the go-ahead, the double bell, and it started up again. In the far distance there was the cry of a youngster calling, probably playing hide-and-seek. For all that I knew, there could be hiding and hunting with me as the quarry now, and newspapers the hunters.

It was nine o'clock. I turned the wireless on. The Home Service news was starting: the Allies weren't going to try Emperor Hirohito as a war criminal; Jewish terrorists had killed two British officers in Palestine; Albert Speer, architect of Hitler's Reich, was beginning his defence at the Nuremberg trials. (Pierrepoint had already hanged thirteen staff of Belsen concentration camp one day, before lunch; it was a pity about Dicky Walters's condition – he'd have appreciated that.) In Belfast an ex-RAF pilot had won his appeal against the death sentence and had been freed. I found Radio Luxemburg, and Sinatra, the new sensation, with his latest hit. It seemed that he needed someone to watch over him.

I was thinking of Mary when the front doorbell rang.

'Greetings, and I hope to Christ you've got plenty of drink in the house,' the Doctor shouted. The Lawyer was next: 'My tongue's stuck to the roof of my bloody mouth.' They pushed past, eyeing their surroundings, calculating drink chances.

Aggie and Dicky were behind them. I put my arms around each in turn. Dicky smiled at Aggie, waiting: she was carrying a book. 'He wants you to have that,' she said. I brought them inside. It was his log book. 'Oh, no.' I shook my head, but Aggie pushed the book back. 'Take it,' she said. Dicky was nodding.

'Thanks very much, old chum.' I held it to my chest. I shoved a hand in my pocket. 'Are you all right for lira?'

Aggie winked: 'We're OK, thanks to the Royal Canadian Navy.' She pushed Dicky to me. I put my arms around him.

'Chocks away, Hughie,' Dicky said. There was no emotion in his voice: he just said it, smiling the same smile he'd worn since he'd come in.

I saw them to the door. 'I'll write to you,' I said, on the step. 'I'll write to you both,' I told Aggie, 'you'll always hear from me.'

They began to walk down the path. 'Chocks away, ou! mate,' I called. Dicky waved. They walked into the light of the street lamp outside, and through the first tears that I'd shed that day, their silhouettes dissolved into a thousand lines and angles, until there was nothing left to distort except the golden light of the lamp. I stood at the door, waited for proper composure to return, then went inside.

The Lawyer and the Doctor had found the drinks cabinet. Their glasses were better than generously filled; I took the whiskey bottle from the Doctor and put it back. 'We were in the crowd outside your flat,' the Doctor said. 'We saw the man calling to see Aggie and Dicky and we rumbled.'

'That's what comes of having a high DQ,' the Lawyer added. 'Drink quotient,' he explained. 'What about your own libation, dear boy? You're improperly dressed; you've no drink.' He slapped my shoulder. 'Thank God to see you back, Hughie; you're the boy'll see us right, for digs and drink, eh?'

'I'm off the broth,' I told them.

They gaped. 'Do you know this?' The Doctor's voice had dropped almost to nothing. 'I feel worse hearing you say that than when they told me you were going to swing.'

'Off the broth?' the Lawyer half-screamed. 'Hugh, old chap, jail has done this to you.'

'Indeed and it has,' I smiled at them both.

'It has left you all bitter and twisted,' the Lawyer said brokenly.

I gave them a last drink, showed them to the door, and they walked away down the road, staying close to each other for comfort. I went back into the quiet room, washed the glasses, put them back, sat down, and thought about the drink.

It had been a bit of a miracle, staying off it through the last hours. But if I could hold it back in times like these, then I could lick it for good. There was no halfway, no kid-stakes about cutting it down. It had to be all the way, or nothing. Curiously enough, thinking about it in those terms, I got the writing tingle. After all those months, it was waking up. I could write, wherever I ended up. My AA experts had said in the Crum that the hardest thing in their newly sober lives had been to find something to fill the space that drinking had taken up. Well, I'd have no problem in that direction. I could write. I loved it. Just before I'd gone into jail my plans were beginning to move on. I'd begun to think about fiction, maybe a play for radio.

The phone rang; it was O'Hare. His voice was careful but welcoming. 'Got your message. Sorry I can't make it across town to see you; I've got to address a union meeting of the night cleaners at Stormont. I'd have come up to see you before, only it's awkward, being a JP and that.'

'Oh, sure. Have they made you a senator yet?'

'There's a set time for that. I'm on course for it, as you would say. But I'm right into the trade-union game. That idea of yours was inspired. I'm lapping it up, I'm running for the executive council next month. I should get the Prod vote.'

I lowered my voice: 'Jesus, Jack, your message really got me going. It was touch and go whether I went crackers or not. I was resigned to the rope, you see. Were you confident?'

There was a pause, then: 'Look, Hughie, you're out, just be content with that . . .' There was another silence. 'Don't you worry about the hows and the whys. But I'll just ask you one thing: don't you agree that things have turned out right, with that left-footer only getting the jail for the same thing?'

Things had turned out right, all right. Squared, and raised to the power of a squillion. O'Hare for King, I waited.

He was talking, low-voiced, but animatedly. 'We have to win everything, or else we lose everything, do you understand? We have to win the big things and the small things, everything. If only a wee tiny crack appears we could lose the lot and then it'll be Christ help the Prods.' I made assenting noises. Finally O'Hare said: 'Hughie, I don't know where you'll be going, but Canada's loyal. I have contacts there. Keep in touch. Bye bye, and mind yourself.'

I made myself a cup of tea. I had just finished drinking it when the doorbell rang: I ran down the hall to answer it.

It was Bill.

I wanted to see him and it was lovely, but I never thought I'd see the day when opening the door and seeing our Bill would leave me disappointed.

'John's out there,' he said quickly. I saw, by the kerb, a black, well-used Hillman Minx. Inside its square body John was sitting over the wheel. Beside him a woman sat; she wore some sort of fine head square, to protect a new perm; she had a light coat over her shoulders. Bill was talking fast. 'He wasn't going to come. The man from the prison came to the house just as they called to see me on their way to some kind of a dinner. John said he didn't want to see you, but hearing he was your brother the man nearly ate him, but it was me that made them come.'

John was getting out of the car. I gestured for Bill to go inside and wait.

I kept my hands to my sides. From the cut of him, there'd be no handshake from John.

'Well,' I said just the one word, a linking word, a bridge between people sharing some kind of experience, but there was no link and no bridge about John's tight mouth, so that side of the argument was settled. He wasn't coming in to talk and he wasn't coming close at the door.

He wore a navy blazer with some sort of badge at the pocket, good grey flannels, a country check shirt and a club tie. On his feet were brown shoes.

'I'm going away for good,' I said.

When he spoke his voice was rough, uneven. 'Good. Sooner the better.' His hair, cut army-short, was clean and shining, his face was windburned, no doubt from golfing. The parade-ground glance took in, with loathing, my wrinkled trousers, unpressed shirt, scuffed shoes, long, unwashed hair, the Crumlin pallor.

He was my brother, and I loved him, but jail had only taken some of the burn from my pepper, it hadn't made dust of it. 'Just as well I'm going,' I said, with the needle smile, 'now maybe you can stick a hyphen on to your name and English yourself to fuck.'

He was biting the inside of his mouth, shaking his head. The right words wouldn't come. He stood, looking me in the eye. 'Bastard.' He said it low and long. Then he turned and walked back to the car.

I beat him to it. I opened the door and said: 'Hello, Annie.'

With her head turned to John and away from me, she said: 'Honest, John, I don't know how you could bring yourself. You know I didn't want to come here.'

John was putting the key in the ignition. He was nodding to his wife, in acknowledgment. I bent over, until she could no longer avoid my eyes. John waited, his eyes narrowing.

'Try to believe this, Annie,' I said, with my face two inches from hers, and her head back against the leather of the seat. 'I didn't want to come here either, and I wouldn't be here, if it hadn't been for something that Leo Grogan said.'

Balls to you, I thought. You're not John: you're not entitled.

Puzzled, John looked from me to his wife, then he turned the key. I watched until the car's bellow faded to a grumble, until the rear lights sank below a dip in the road opposite the Catholic chapel, and I still stood, until there was no sound but the far murmur of the city and the whisper of the evening wind in the lime trees.

I went in to see my kid brother. He was more able to control himself, more the man now, with filled-out shoulders and a shaving track, but, in his blue innocent eyes worry still showed about my going. We talked, and as we did, I listened all the time for the doorbell.

'How are you getting on, in the house on your own?' I asked him.

'For dear sake, I can't move for women. Aunt Nell lands in with grub in saucepans and the wives on each side of me keep giving me cake and dumpling.'

'You'll need to watch yourself. You're a bit of a catch, now, with a house and all. The girls'll be after you.' By his smile, it had already started. 'I'll always keep in touch,' I told Bill. 'You know, we could meet, wherever you end up. I'm going to sea when I finish my time, don't forget.'

'That'll be some reunion, eh?'

Hating to do it, I hurried the farewells. 'Mary might call,' I told Bill. I wanted to mention her name.

'I hope she does,' he said, and I felt uneasy at the lack of certainty.

'I sent a message to her,' I went on, still wanting to talk about her. 'Maybe she was out when it was left, but it'll be in her hall when she gets back.'

'Write plenty of letters,' Bill said. I promised, and watched him go down the road, slowly, with his head down.

When he'd gone I closed the door, went inside, and sat down to listen. After a few minutes I jumped up and turned off the wireless, even though it had only been playing softly. I didn't want anything to cover the sound of the bell. I even opened the door into the hall, to give it every chance.

My hands were being squeezed tight between my knees, and I sat well forward, straining, in the way that I'd sat for so many long hours on the edge of my prison bed. I kept raising each heel in turn from the ground, to make the flat palms of my hands rub together.

When the bell rang, even after all my preparations, I found that I couldn't rush to answer it. I just sat there, in the prison way, rubbing my hands between my knees.

After half a minute, it rang again. I rose then, slowly walked down the hall, and, almost timorously, turned the lock and opened the door.